TESTING THE WATERS
Lessons from the History of Drug Research

What can we learn from the past that may be relevant to modern drug research?

In this book Allan Gaw shows us how the past can illuminate the present and help us understand where we are and how we have come to be here. We will start in a world, more than two thousand years ago, long before science, but where highly disciplined minds could still formulate rigorous strategies for the evaluation of new drugs. We will move forward to see the parts played by an Emperor's physician in Ancient Rome, a Persian philosopher and a country doctor in England. We will visit the battlefields of Europe, the laboratory benches of a German drug company and see the parts played by serendipity and innovation in the development of new drugs. In the early 20th century we will see that tragedy can be the result of inadequate testing of medicines as well as being the catalyst for change. And, we will discover how the story of one sleeping tablet changed everything.

Allan Gaw, MD, PhD, FRCPath, FFPM, PGCert Med Ed is a Scottish writer and educator. He has been a clinical academic for over 25 years. Most recently, he was Professor & Director of the Clinical Research Facility at Queen's University Belfast, and he previously worked at the University of Glasgow and UT Southwestern in Dallas, Texas.

In addition to over 25 books, he also writes articles on a range of subjects and a blog entitled *The Business of Discovery* (researchet.wordpress.com). If you would like to learn more about him and his work, visit his website www.allangaw.com or follow him on twitter @ResearchET.

i

SELECTED OTHER WORKS

Gaw A. *Tales from an Oxford Bench.* SA Press, Glasgow 2014.

Gaw A. *WriteEasy: A Strategy for More Effective Scientific Writing.* SA Press, Glasgow, 2014.

Gaw A. *WordEasy: The Commonest Grammatical Mistakes in Formal Writing & How to Avoid Them.* SA Press, Glasgow, 2013.

Gaw A. *SpeakEasy: 7 Ingredients for Effective Presentations.* SA Press, Glasgow, 2012.

Gaw A. *Abstract Expressions – A Quick Guide to Writing Effective Abstracts for Conferences and Papers.* SA Press, Glasgow, 2011.

Gaw A and Burns MHJ. *On Moral Grounds – Lessons from the History of Research Ethics.* SA Press, Glasgow, 2011.

Gaw A. *Our Speaker Today – A Guide to Effective Lecturing.* SA Press, Glasgow, 2010.

Gaw A. *Trial by Fire – Lessons from the History of Clinical Trials.* SA Press, Glasgow, 2009.

TESTING THE WATERS
Lessons from the History of Drug Research

Allan Gaw, MD, PhD

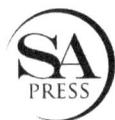

SA PRESS

First published 2016

by SA Press

SAPress42@gmail.com

© 2016 Allan Gaw

British Library Cataloguing in Publication Data

A catalogue record for this book is available from the British Library.

ISBN 13: 978-0-9563242-5-2

For those who ask why it is so difficult

...it is better the world should derive some instruction, however imperfect, from my experience, than that the lives of men should be hazarded by its unguarded exhibition, or that a medicine of so much efficacy should be condemned and rejected as dangerous and unmanageable.

William Withering, 1785

An Account of the Foxglove and Some of its Medical Uses

··■··

The investigation of drugs is a task for the pharmacologist and not for a chemist or pharmacist, who until now have been expected to do this. We have to be acquainted with the tools which we use. The appearance of Senna leaves is a matter of indifference to the pharmacologist, just as it is unimportant for the surgeon what the box looks like from which he selects the scalpels for an operation. However, it is important which constituents determine the action of Senna leaves, and what are their properties; likewise, it cannot be irrelevant whether the box contains instruments suitable for dissection or not, and where the backs and the cutting edges of the knives are. Fortunately, a surgeon who uses the wrong side of the scalpel cuts his own fingers and not the patient; if the same applied to drugs, they would have been investigated very carefully a long time ago...

Rudolf Buchheim, 1849

Beitrage zur Arzneimittellehre

CONTENTS

FOREWORD

Sir William Osler is regarded by many as the father of modern medicine and he made many contributions both to the study and teaching of his subject. One of his observations is especially pertinent to the topic of this book. He drew a fundamental distinction between humans and beasts when he noted in 1891:

> A desire to take medicine is, perhaps, the great feature which distinguishes man from other animals.

Modern medicine, and indeed modern life, is difficult to imagine without the ready availability of well-researched and effective medications, but think for a moment: what would our world look like if there were no drug treatments?

First, the global population, which has recently passed the 7 billion mark would be less — considerably less. Deaths from many diseases, but especially infectious diseases would be high. In consequence, the population would be on average much younger, for the likelihood of reaching old age would be much reduced. The average number of pregnancies for each woman would be much higher as infant mortality would be high, as of course would be rates of maternal death in childbirth. Pain would be unrelieved, infections untreated, psychiatric diseases unresolved. Patients with diabetes could expect nothing like a normal life. Children with asthma would struggle and many would die from their condition. Sexually transmitted diseases would be rife and often ultimately fatal. There would be greater dependency on folk remedies and alternative therapies — only they would no longer be alternative, but mainstream.

Medicine as a professional discipline would also look very different: built less upon a scientific foundation and more upon an unstable and shifting edifice of opinion and belief and faith.

We should not have to work too hard to imagine this world for it *was* our world in the comparatively recent past. The explosion in drug development has largely been a story written in the last two or three centuries and this narrative has been driven by many different factors. Yes, there have been commercial interests but there has also been a genuine desire to improve the health of the population and to relieve suffering. Lofty words that lose a little of their altitude when we think of drug scandals and the deception and greed of some academic and commercial groups, but words that are nonetheless true. The development of new drugs has often been driven in the first instance by a simple wish to help, and not merely to make money. Successful drugs will make enormous wealth for those who develop and manufacture them, but the pharmaceutical business is also a very risky and expensive one, as we shall see. Huge speculative investment must be made to find and test the next novel compound. Many, if not most, contenders will fall by the wayside and only a tiny minority of new compounds will eventually find their way on to the pharmacy shelves. But, it was not always so.

As we will see, as we explore the history of this subject, the regulation of drug development is comparatively new and was often enacted as a response to scandal or catastrophe. Similarly, the scientific rigour applied to drug development and testing is also a relatively modern phenomenon. However, modern medicine does not have a monopoly on innovation, and there is evidence of an ethical and responsible approach to research in the past. If we look hard enough, we can find the concepts central to modern drug development on the pages of ancient treatises. But, while we can point to many moments of creativity and excellence we can also identify practices that would not only offend our modern sensibilities, but scandalise them.

This book, like the two others in the series, takes as its basic premise that there is something of worth to be learned by examining the past. In his recent book, *A History of 20th Century Britain*, Andrew Marr notes, 'History is either a moral argument with lessons for the here-and-now or it is merely an accumulation of pointless facts.'

This is not always immediately obvious, and certainly if we look at the more than two thousand years of history covered by the stories in this book, we may reasonably question its truth. But, I believe firmly that by entering these worlds from the past, by studying them and analysing them, we do come away richer and better equipped to understand the present. When it comes to pharmaceutical research, the present is a complex scientific, legal and regulatory maze that has evolved across the world to protect patients; by assuring the quality of drugs, the rigour of their testing and the balance of their safety and effectiveness.

I do not aim to offer a comprehensive history of drug research, for to do so would require many volumes. Instead, I want to tell the story of this remarkable aspect of human endeavour by focusing on a number of pivotal moments during the last few thousand years. Inevitably, this means that I have been selective in what I present but in each case I have chosen carefully to highlight what I believe to be the key moments and the principal players in this story.

We will begin more than two thousand years ago in a world long before science, but where highly disciplined minds could still formulate rigorous strategies for the evaluation of new drugs. We will move through the centuries and witness the development of medicine and clinical research. We will see the parts played by an Emperor's physician in Ancient Rome, a Persian philosopher and a country doctor in England. We will visit the battlefields of Europe and the laboratory benches of a German drug company and see the hands of both serendipity and innovation at work in the development of new drugs. Moving on to the beginnings of what we might regard as modern medicine in the 18ᵗʰ century we will look at the discovery and testing of one of the first pharmaceuticals. At the dawn of the 20th century we will see that tragedy can be the result of inadequate regulation and the catalyst for change. As we move into living memory we will see the consequences of inadequate pre-clinical and clinical testing of new drugs and discover how the story of one sleeping tablet changed everything.

In each case we can enjoy the narrative as an interesting historical vignette, but these stories are included for more than simple entertainment. Each teaches us a lesson that is relevant and resonant today. For the most part these stories are about people long dead, from other worlds, but we should not forget that they were in many ways no different from ourselves. They were adults and children, healthy and sick, good and bad. What happened in each case, like a pebble tossed into a lake, sent ripples across the years. Those ripples still lap against the shores of the present, inviting us to catch them, dipping our fingers and testing the waters.

———— ■ ————

ACKNOWLEDGMENTS

At a Christmas party at couple of years ago, I was asked by a friend what I hoped to achieve in the coming year. Without hesitation, but admittedly soothed by my host's good cheer, I said I wanted to write another book on the history of medicine. He looked back at me and in silence threw a gauntlet at my feet. The book would be the third in a series. Each volume has been progressively harder to write, not because there is less to say, but because there is more.

Researching the history of my subject has opened many new doors and introduced me to new colleagues and friends, who have taught me that there is always more to learn, to understand and to share. Without the encouragement of these individuals, without the enthusiasm of my readers for the previous two books in this series and without that gauntlet, which I picked up, I doubt if this book would have been written.

I must also acknowledge the debts I owe to those who have kindly read and commented on early drafts of the following chapters. Despite their valuable input I emphasise, however, that any factual errors or pieces of clumsy prose that remain are entirely my own.

I must also thank other individuals and organizations for various acts of kindness that helped with researching of the topics, the sourcing of illustrations or the production of the book.

    SJ Littleford — for helping me access key literature in Oxford.

    Alexander A Gaw and Thomas Demant — for helping me with the translations of Reil's and Nolde's rules from the original German.

David Tolmie — for help with the cover design.

The University of Birmingham Research and Cultural Collections — for allowing me to reproduce the portrait of William Withering.

While every effort has been made to identify the copyright holders of the photographs used in the book, several have remained elusive. If you hold the copyright of any unattributed image, please contact me and I will ensure this is corrected in any subsequent edition of the book.

Finally, I would like to thank my editor at SA Press, Moira Mungall, who creates with apparent effortlessness such a creative environment in which to work and provides much needed encouragement and support at every step of the way.

——— ■ ———

I

Poisoned Arrows and Venetian Treacle

The Beginnings of Medicine

Introduction

To speak of beginnings suggests there was one. When it comes to 'medicine', however, it is hard to imagine there was ever a time when people were uninterested in their health; that there was ever a time when they were not concerned with healing or the possibility of easing pain or calming fever. In short, it is difficult to imagine a time when we did not resort to the use of drugs. Of course, to use such a modern term as 'drugs' is misleading for our distant ancestors had no notion of specific chemicals with pharmacological actions on the body, or their interactions with metabolic and cellular processes.

Despite this lack of specific knowledge of drug action, which is a very recent development, our ancestors would have known a thing or two about what would happen if you ate the wrong berry, or used the wrong leaf or tree sap to soothe a wound. This knowledge may have been handed down through generations, mixed with magic and superstition, but it must have originated in observation. Our ancestors would have watched what happened when one of their clan suffered and died after eating the leaves of the deadly nightshade or the foxglove. They would have watched the toxic effects of the scorpion's sting and the adder's bite. They had the wit to find a cause and effect in the sequence of these events and this, perhaps taken together with other similar observations, would be induced into a principle — that plant is bad for you; that snake should be avoided.

At what point this principle was first turned on its head and the knowledge used, not to prevent harm, but to cause it, is unknown. However, it was not long before people discovered the power of the toxins in their environment, and used this knowledge for hunting or even homicide. Nor would it be long before they would also find therapeutic uses for the large and diverse pharmacy that nature had to offer.

Toxicology, the study of poisons, is probably where it began, for simple, practical reasons. The poisonous plants, animals and minerals of the ancient world were, by necessity, well known to cavemen. If they weren't our ancestors would have died, by eating the wrong things. Even the Garden of Eden had a snake, and it probably also had a few plants that would have given Adam and Eve more than a dose of knowledge. But as the 16th century Swiss physician Paracelsus noted: 'Poison is in everything, and no thing is without poison. The dosage makes it either a poison or a remedy.' This is often abbreviated to the aphorism: 'The dose makes the poison' and serves to remind us that there is always a very fine line between toxicology and therapeutics.

Prehistoric beginnings

It is believed that 10-20 thousand years ago, as man developed stone tipped arrows for hunting, they also dreamt up the idea of dipping them in poison — just to make sure. (fig. 1.1) Indeed, the term toxicology is derived from the Greek word *toxikon*, which means a bow with which to shoot poisoned arrows or the poison itself into which the arrowheads are dipped. (1) Various primitive societies around the world developed such arrow poisons and some are still used today — curare is one of the toxins of choice in South America, while in Africa they prefer ouabain. Both these poisons are also used therapeutically in modern medicine — curare and its derivatives in anaesthesia, and ouabain and the cardiac glycosides derived from it in cardiology.

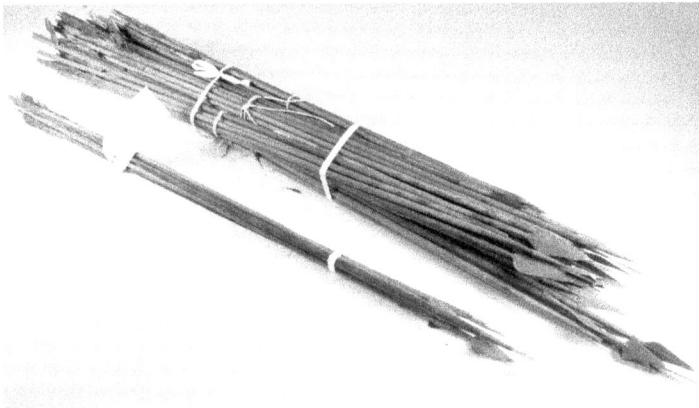

Figure 1.1. Bundle of 20th century poisoned arrows collected in the Democratic Republic of the Congo (CC Attribution: Brooklyn Museum).

Thus, the necessary 'experimental' work that would allow such poisons to be avoided or used safely was probably completed many millennia ago. Of course, we know nothing of the details of these investigations as no records of such fieldwork or experiments exist. Things only start to get written down when we invent writing. The 'we' in question were the Sumerians, who lived in modern day Iraq, and it is thought that the first cuneiform texts were inscribed around 3,000 BCE. Thus, people are known to have used medicinal plants, such as liquorice, mustard, myrrh, and opium from at least 5,000 BCE and the oldest extant Mesopotamian medical text is a therapeutic manual written in Sumerian and dating from around 2,100 BCE. (fig. 1.2) (2) However, that text written on clay tablets is likely to be a version of earlier texts of almost 1,000 years before. This is true of most of the contenders for the earliest pharmacopoeias: in each case the earliest tablet or scroll we have is probably only a copy of an even earlier text or a transcription of an even earlier oral tradition.

Fast forward a thousand years or so and we meet the ancient Egyptians, an advanced civilisation in many ways who, like the Sumerians, recognised the need to document their own pharmacopoeia. Various Egyptian papyri have been uncovered and translated, most notably the Ebers Papyrus, named after the German Egyptologist who offered the first translation of the work. (fig. 1.3) (3) That papyrus dates from c1,550 BCE, but contains writings copied from much older texts, possibly as early as 3,000 BCE. This, the longest of the ancient Egyptian medical papyri, includes, as well as descriptions of human anatomy and physiology, over 800 prescriptions, which take the form of 'salves, plasters, and poultices; snuffs, inhalations, and gargles; draughts, confections, and pills; fumigations, suppositories, and enemata.' (3) Many of these are simple concoctions, with just a single component, but others are much more complex and one has as many as 37 ingredients.

These prescriptions include some that would be familiar to us today, such as aloe vera for skin complaints, mint to aid digestion and poppy to deaden pain. But, amongst these remedies you will also find a mixture of magic and wishful-thinking. While raw meat is suggested as a treatment for a black eye, other treatments, we are instructed, should only be taken while seated cross-legged or after sexual intercourse, and some of the raw ingredients might raise a modern eyebrow, such as 'water-in-which-the phallus-has-been-washed'.

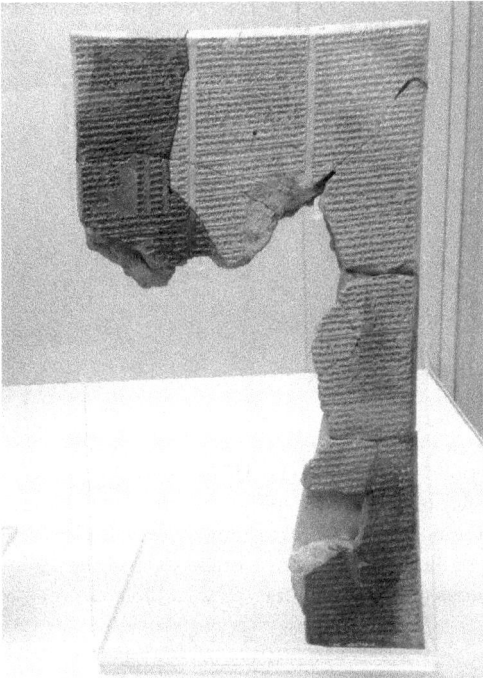

Figure 1.2. A six-column clay tablet containing prescriptions and spells written in Sumerian. Each section contains a list of drugs and instructions for their use (British Museum, Photo by the author).

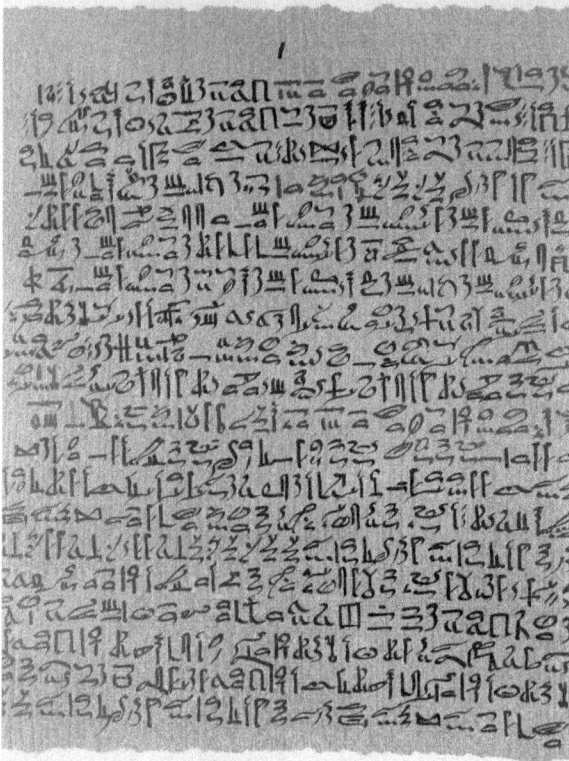

Figure 1.3. Found in Egypt in the 1870s, the *Ebers Papyrus* contains prescriptions written in hieroglyphics for over 800 remedies. This details a prescription for an asthma remedy, which is to be prepared as a mixture of herbs heated on a brick so that the patient could inhale their fumes (Wellcome Library/Public Domain).

Shen Nung

These Sumerian and Egyptian writings may be the roots of a Western medical tradition, but on the other side of the globe ancient Chinese medicine was flourishing and being documented at around the same time. One candidate as the father of Chinese medicine (and there are many) was Emperor Shen Nung. (4) He is believed to have lived and reigned around 2,800 BCE, and as well as introducing the art of acupuncture to the Chinese people, legend tells us that he was the author of the Pen T'sao or native herbal. (fig. 1.4) And the legend specifically states that of the 365 herbal preparations in his pharmacopoeia he tried them all personally. Shen Nung was an empiricist then, even if he was a self-experimenter.

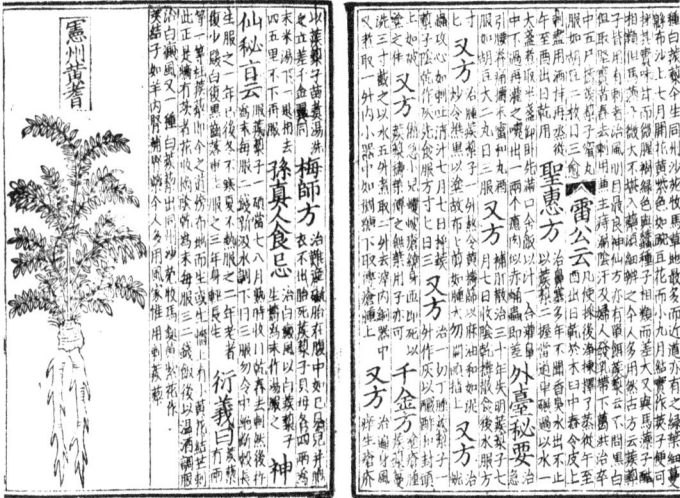

Figure 1.4. Shen Nung Pen T'sao Mid 13th century woodblock (Public Domain)

Dioscorides

It would take the West almost 3,000 years to catch up with Chinese herbalism, but when it did it would again be through the work of an individual who believed in empiricism and fieldwork rather than hearsay.

Pedianos Dioscorides was a doctor in the Roman army. (5) Of Greek origins, he was born in modern day Turkey in 40 CE. He became a physician and his active service in several parts of the Empire facilitated his travel and fed his appetite for botanical knowledge, for Dioscorides was first and foremost a medical herbalist. He saw the therapeutic power, as well as the toxic potential, in the diverse flora of the Roman Empire.

He collected specimens, carefully observing their structure and habitat and, rather than rely on folklore, he recorded their effects through personal experience. His friend and fellow physician Areius urged him to write about his findings and Dioscorides obliged with a five volume work in Greek that has largely become known by its Latinised name, *De Materia Medica*. (fig. 1.5) In this work, written about 70 CE, he describes around a thousand remedies including approximately 600 plants or plant products.

In his dedication to Areius, Dioscorides is dismissive of some physicians, whom he refers to as mere 'poets'. He goes on to write,

> In a way they have condescended to describe commonplace information familiar to all but they have explained the strengths of medicines and their properties briefly, not considering their value by personal experience, but by worthless discussion created needless controversy regarding each medicine, and in addition they have mistakenly recorded one thing for another. (5)

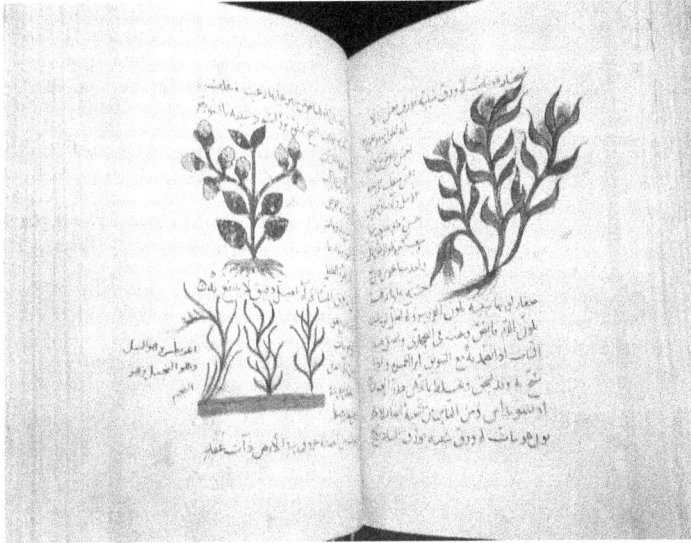

Figure 1.5. Pages from an Arabic edition of Dioscorides' *De Materia Medica* possibly created in Baghdad in c1240. This 13th century copy, like many other versions of *De Materia Medica*, contains many images of plants and herbs, suggesting that the original, now lost, was similarly profusely illustrated (Bodleian Library, Oxford. Photo by the author).

He is particularly disparaging of those whom he feels have perpetuated errors through their lack of empirical knowledge, and of one in particular he states,

> ... and in the face of contradictory evidence he reports an abundance of untruths, which proves that he obtained his information from erroneous gossip, not from personal experience. (5)

Although he undoubtedly used information from other ancient texts, Dioscorides' book was largely written on the basis of extensive fieldwork and it remained the authority on the subject in the West for the next 1,600 years.

Attalus III of Pergamon

But, Shen Nung and Dioscorides were not the only ancient herbalists who realised that experimental evidence rather than folklore must be relied upon, especially when it came to toxicology. In the second century BCE, King Attalus III Philometor of Pergamon, a city-state now in modern Turkey, was famed for his disinterest in politics and his obsession with poisonous plants. (6) These, he carefully cultivated in his gardens, and tested them with their putative antidotes on prisoners condemned to death. This justification of potentially life-threatening clinical experimentation on those already scheduled to die was not unique to the ancient world, but it was a point that drew praise from Attalus' biographers. He is also described as a mad man with a dishevelled appearance and unruly hair and beard, who delighted in sending posies of deadly plants to his friends. All this may, however, have been contemporary propaganda to paint him as an unsuitable figure to rule. Indeed, on his death, without any heirs, he bequeathed his entire kingdom to the Senate and people of Rome, perhaps to avoid a civil war.

As a king, his fascination with toxicology is not unique in the ancient world, where coups were often acted out through the stealthily administered phial of poison. Just after Attalus III died, a boy was born who would become the King of Pontus and who some have named the 'Poison King'. (6)

Mithridates VI of Pontus

King Mithridates VI Eupator of Pontus, a large kingdom around the Black Sea, partly in modern day Turkey, Ukraine, Russia, Romania, Bulgaria and Georgia, lived from 120-63 BCE. (7) His father was assassinated by poison and he spent his life searching for a universal antidote for his own protection. After studying all known poisons, venoms and their antidotes he created a cocktail of all those that were effective. He is reputed to have taken a daily prophylactic dose of his own formula and to have successfully staved off any poisoning attempts. This universal antidote is named after him — Mithridatium — and although it was reconfigured regularly it survived in one form or another for the next 2,000 years.

Mithridates was an experimentalist and, like his predecessor Atallus III, he chose to test his poisons and their antidotes on condemned men. Criminals awaiting their executions were doubtless given little choice on whether they took part in the King's clinical research. But, in addition to being his research subjects, these unfortunates were also part of the after dinner entertainment.

Mithridates, as well as being a researcher, was a showman who would amaze his banquetting guests with demonstrations of the effects of poisons on the human body and would show his own immunity by sampling a variety of toxins — even drinking the venom of deadly snakes. His guests would be astonished by the stark comparison of their host's survival and the demise of his hapless research subjects.

Mithridates VI was also one of the Roman Empire's arch enemies and successfully took on its greatest generals and their armies. When his luck ran out, he chose a more honourable exit than capture, and legend has it that when he tried to commit suicide by self-poisoning he was unable to do so because of the tolerance he had developed over the years by his own use of mithridatium. When his suicide pill failed, he had no alternative but to turn to his bodyguard and seek the help of his strong right arm. The bodyguard obliged and Mithridates died by the sword.

Mithridatium and Theriac

When Pontus fell, the King's experimental notes were seized and returned to Rome. The original mithridatium contained around 46 ingredients including opium, ginger, saffron and castor. Over a century later Andromachus, Emperor Nero's personal physician, reformulated the mithridatium and increased its ingredient list to 64, including mashed viper's flesh. This variant of mithridatium that included components of poisonous reptiles, became known as theriac. (fig. 1.6) This term is derived from the Greek *theria*, which means wild animals. Another century later, Galen, the person physician of Emperor Marcus Aurelius, was a great exponent of theriac and even wrote an entire book devoted to its uses. His Emperor was also reputed to take daily doses of the cocktail.

Theriac is thought to have taken 40 days to prepare after which it was allowed to mature. Galen, himself, recommended that this be for 12 years. This extensive preparation meant that theriac, like the finest single malts, was an expensive luxury available only to the rich.

By the 12th century theriac was being manufactured almost exclusively in Venice from where it was exported throughout the known world. In England, it became known as Venetian Treacle—the latter being a corruption of the word theriac. (8) Indeed, it would not be until the 1690s that we would use the word *treacle*, as we do today, for molasses.

While theriac undoubtedly contained a range of pharmacologically active components, such as opium, it was not, nor could it be, the panacea that everyone thought. Little empirical work was carried out to establish its efficacy or otherwise and when it failed to cure or protect it was considered to be a consequence of its defective manufacture rather than its innate uselessness. Its preparation, therefore, became a matter of public scrutiny and the manufacture of theriac attracted considerable pomp and ceremony throughout the centuries. (fig. 1.7) Indeed, even in 1722 it was still being publicly and ceremoniously prepared by the London Society of Apothecaries and sold in pots stamped with their seal.

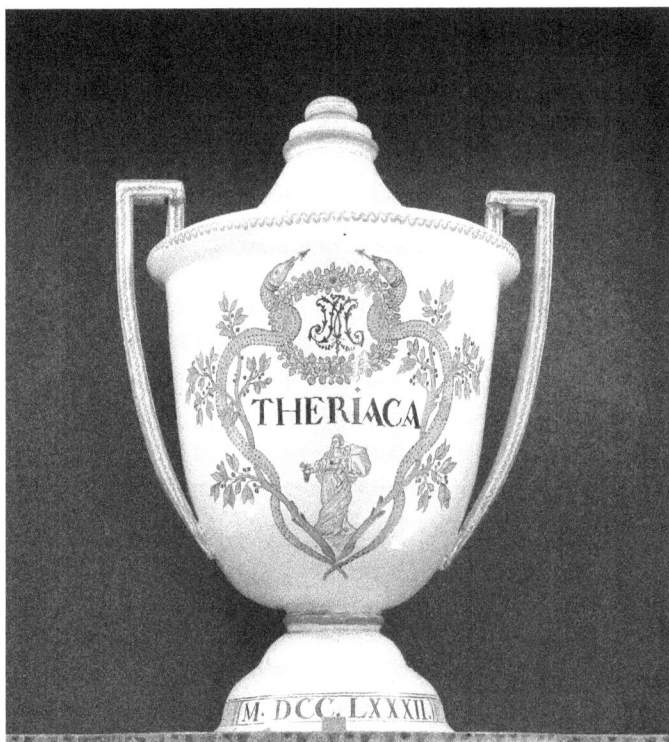

Figure 1.6. 18th Century Theriac Jar, from the Pharmacie des Hospices de Beaune, France (CC Attribution: Jebulon).

The development of pharmaceutical regulation also owes its origins to these quality concerns. (9) In the reign of Henry VIII, the Pharmacy Wares, Drugs and Stuffs Act of 1540 was

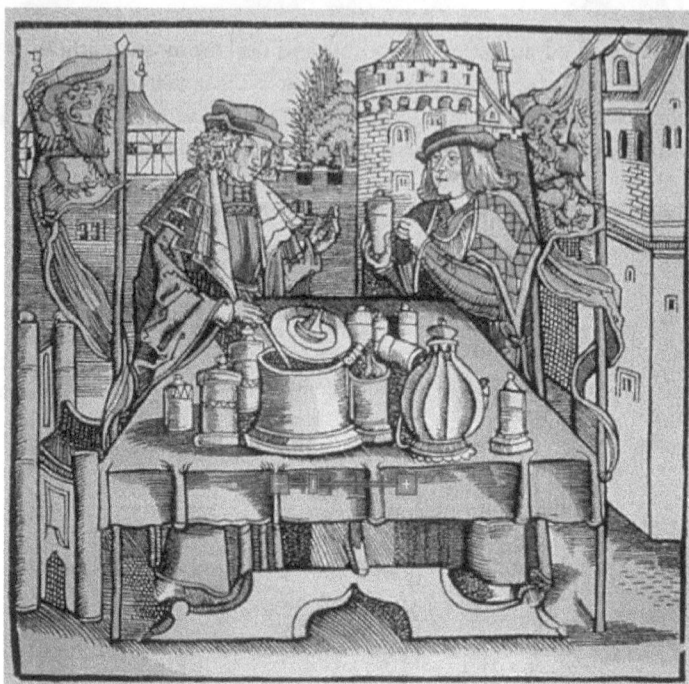

Figure 1.7. Woodcut showing the public preparation of the theriac in Strasbourg in 1537 [Courtesy of Images from the History of Medicine (NLM): Public Domain].

passed, which controlled the manufacture of theriac, and in the reign of Elizabeth I, only a single apothecary, William Besse, was authorised to make mithridatium, which was then subject to inspection by the Royal College of Physicians.

Recipes for mithridatium and theriac found their way into the new pharmacopoeias of the early modern era and in 1665, when the Great Plague was at its height, these remedies were regarded as the definitive treatment for the disease. Concerns about the quality of these panaceas continued and statuary inspections of apothecary shops, which had begun in Henry VIII's reign continued, throughout the 17th, 18th and early 19th centuries. Commonly it was the quality and composition of the Venetian (or by now London) Treacle, theriac or mithridatium that were called into question.

The beginning of the end for these preparations was in 1745 when the English physician William Heberden (fig. 1.8) published a 19-page pamphlet entitled: Antitheriaca, An Essay on Mithridatium and Theriaca. (fig. 1.9) In this work, he quotes Pliny, whom he describes as an authority 'almost as old as the Theriaca' and who 'declaims with great vehemence against the injudiciousness, the ostentation and wantonness of this heap of drugs'. He also refers to the mystery surrounding its manufacture: 'it still goes on to be prepared in the old manner as near as maybe in all the great cities of Europe'.

Heberden notes that the value of theriac and mithridatium rests largely on the ancient authority with which they have come down to us, but questions the veracity of these claims. He also states, 'Experience alone can be called in to vouch for its character, and no better voucher can be desired; but experience is clearly against it.' However, without any real experimental evidence, Heberden goes on to argue his case through an historical analysis: 'There cannot surely be a stronger proof of a medicine's insignificancy, than its losing ground so remarkably after a tryal of near two thousand years with a constant prepossession in its favour.'

As well as questioning the efficacy of theriac and mithridatium, Heberden raised concerns about its safety. While he believed the principal effective component of these concoctions was opium he noted that, because of the highly variable recipes used, the amounts of opium administered may be equally variable and potentially fatal. He was also more generally concerned with the impact of polypharmacy when he concluded that this is a 'medley of discordant Simples . . . made up of a dissonant crowd collected from different countries, mighty in appearance, but in reality, an ineffective multitude that only hinder one another.'

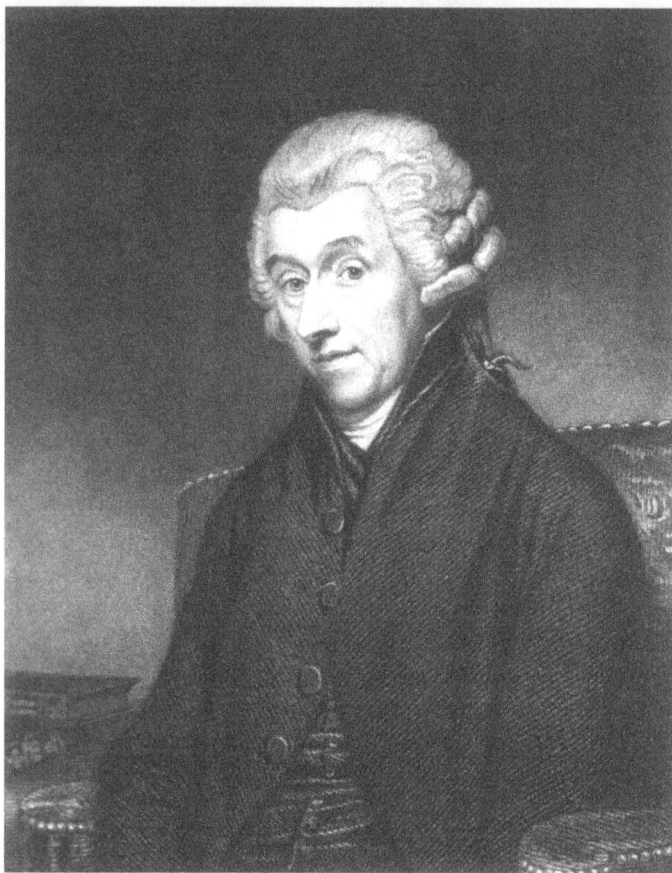

Figure 1.8. William Heberden (1710-1801) [Courtesy of Images from the History of Medicine (NLM): Public Domain].

The London Pharmacopoeia dropped the recipes for mithridatium and theriac from its 1788 edition, while the Edinburgh Pharmacopeia had seen the light a little earlier and their 1756 edition was panacea free. However, recipes for these ancient, composite remedies could still be found in the German Pharmacopoeia of 1872 and its French counterpart as late as 1884, and it was still available for purchase in Rome a century later.

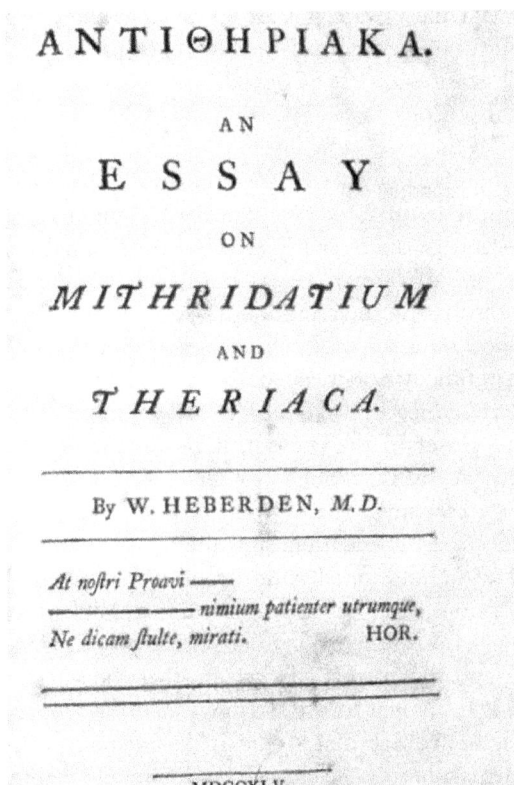

ΑΝΤΙΘΗΡΙΑΚΑ.

AN

E S S A Y

ON

MITHRIDATIUM

AND

THERIACA.

By W. HEBERDEN, *M.D.*

At noſtri Proavi ———
——————————— *nimium patienter utrumque,*
Ne dicam ſtulte, mirati.   HOR.

MDCCXLV.

Figure 1.9. Title page of *Antitheriaca. An Essay on Mithridatium and Theriaca* by William Heberden. The partial Latin quotation is from Horace's *Ars Poetica* and translates approximately as, 'But our ancestors praised...too accepting and foolish, then, their admiration.' (Public Domain).

Conclusions

The first 20,000 years of drug research does not, in truth, involve much research, or at least the kind of ordered activity we think of as research today. But it did nonetheless involve meticulous observation and the induction of general and often life-saving principles. As cavemen and women, we had our senses of smell and taste to guide us away from the ingestion of poisons, but these were not always reliable and it was only through painful observation of the effects of our environment on our well-being and that of our kin that we could work out the effects of poisons.

Even in antiquity, however, some recognised the need for a more empirical approach. We have seen the use of self-experimentation to discover the effects of medicinal herbs, as well as the use of human research subjects to evaluate the effects of poisons and their antidotes — and all more than two millennia ago. Human curiosity, coupled with the necessary rigorous experimentation needed to provide answers are far from modern concerns. However, as we move along the timeline and closer to the present, it is sometimes surprising how much we were willing to take for granted, even comparatively recently. For example, the antique provenance of the recipes for mithridatium and theriac seemed to confer upon them an unquestioned faith that today seems unjustified and frankly nonsensical. That it took almost 2,000 years for a physician to seriously question their efficacy is at once both bewildering and remarkable. However, that the question was raised at all is testament to the growing scientific scepticism of a more enlightened age that would make further advances in clinical pharmacology possible. In subsequent chapters, we will see some of the fruits of that enlightenment.

As we began to question and adopt a more rigorous approach to the study of both new and established treatments, we enter a new chapter of our scientific history. Superstition gives way to logic, and supposition yields to the strength of hard evidence. Ultimately, we will see the development of the modern pharmaceutical medico-industrial complex that, in the 20th century, becomes the incubator of many new drugs. But before that there is much work that needs to be done.

References

1. Watson KD, Wexler P and Everitt JM. *History* In: Wexler P, Hakkinen PJ, Kennedy G, Stoss FW (Eds) *Information Resources in Toxicology*, 3rd Ed. Academic Press, San Diego, 2000.

2. Scurlock J, Andersen BR. *Diagnoses in Assyrian and Babylonian Medicine*. University of Illinois Press, Champaign, 2005.

3. Bryan, CP. The Papyrus Ebers. Geoffrey Bles, London 1930.

4. Unschuld PU. *Medicine in China: A History of Pharmaceutics* University of California Press, Berkley, 1986.

5. Osbaldeston TA, Wood RPA. *Dioscorides: De Material Medica (a new indexed version in modern English)*. Ibidis Press, Johannesburg, 2000.

6. Scarborough J. Attalus III of Pergamon research toxicologist. In: Cilliers L (ed) *Asklepios: Studies on Ancient Medicine*. Bloemfontein: Classical Association of South Africa (Acta Classica Supplementum II), 2008, pp. 138-156. http://www.academia.edu/2368049/Attalus_III_of_Pergamon_Research_Toxicologist_2008_ (Accessed 8 January 2016).

7. Mayor A. *The Poison King: The Life and Legend of Mithradates, Rome's Deadliest Enemy*. Princeton University Press, Princeton, 2009.

8. Penn RG. The state control of medicines: the first 3000 years. *British Journal of Clinical Pharmacology* 1979; 8: 293-305.

9.   Griffin JP. Venetian treacle and the foundation of medicines regulation *British Journal of Clinical Pharmacology* 2004; 58: 317-325.

10.   Heberden W. Antitherica — an essay on Mithridatium and Theriaca. Bound in *Royal College of Physicians Transactions* 1745; 112 no. 6.

——— ∎ ———

2

The Burning of Books

The Beginnings of Science

Introduction

In the first chapter, we pondered whether the beginnings of medicine could be pinpointed at all. Might we have any more success with the beginnings of science? Surely, there we are on more solid ground. There must have been a time when we did not seek to discover new knowledge, whether about drugs or any other topic, with anything approaching the scientific method.

Trial and error, superstition and good luck were probably the main drivers of drug discovery and use in pre-history. But, we certainly do not have to wait until the modern era, as some may imagine, to find an appreciation of the value of experimentation and personal experience over folklore.

As good a place as any to begin our search for the beginnings of science is on one summer evening in 1527, when two of the physicians we mentioned in passing in Chapter 1 came together across a gap of fourteen centuries. These were the Roman physician Galen and the Swiss physician Paracelsus.

Paracelsus

Paracelsus, or more correctly Theophrastus Phillippus Aureolus Bombastus von Hohenheim, was a controversial and outspoken critic of ancient medical authority. (fig. 2.1) His teaching methods were unorthodox, e.g. inviting the general public to his lectures, which he delivered in German rather than Latin, while wearing an alchemist's leather apron rather than an academic gown. His medical practice was also unconventional and owed more to his travels and his personal experiences than the accepted medical books of the day. On this, he wrote,

> Wherever I went I eagerly and diligently investigated and sought after the tested and reliable arts of medicine. I went not only to the doctors but also the barbers, bathkeepers, learned physicians, women, and magicians who pursue the art of healing; I went to monasteries, to noble and common folk, to the experts and the simple. (1,2)

Despite the fact that he rejected much of traditional medical knowledge in favour of personal experience through experimentation, he firmly believed in gnomes, spirits and fairies, and there is no evidence that he ever studied medicine in any formal academic institution. (3)

In 1526, he had been appointed to the Chair of Medicine at the University of Basel, Switzerland. However, he was not a popular choice. His arrogance preceded him and many of his contemporaries found him loathsome. But, Paracelsus was undaunted, writing,

> Let me tell you this: every little hair on my neck knows more than you and all your scribes, and my shoebuckles are more learned than your Galen and Avicenna, and my beard has more experience than all your high colleges. (1)

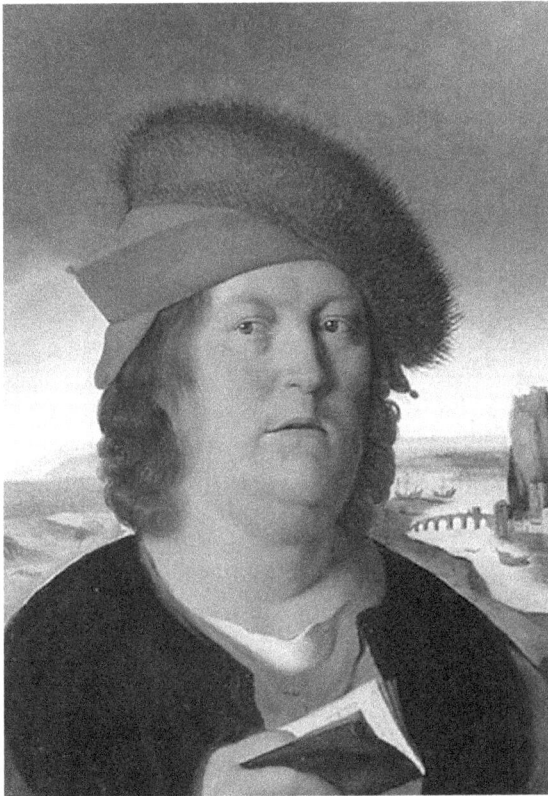

Figure 2.1. Paracelsus (1493-1541) Portion of one of numerous 17th Century copies of an original by Quentin Massys. (CC Attribution: Dake)

Perhaps driven by this arrogance, Paracelsus is reputed to have committed an act of vandalism before the university on St David's Day, 24 June 1527, when, in a show of bravado and iconoclasm, he cast the prized works of Galen and Avicenna into a bonfire. A year later he was thrown out of Basel and he spent his final years as an itinerant, dying in Austria in 1541.

Thomas Percival, an English physician and pioneering medical ethicist of the late 18th century, pulled no punches when he retold the story,

> In the beginning of the sixteenth century, Paracelsus a native of Switzerland stood forth, and with matchless arrogance, and the most supercilious contempt of others, proclaimed his opinions to the world. Seated in his Professorial chair at Basil [sic], he solemnly burnt the writings of Galen and Avicenna, intending to become himself, the sole oracle in physick. But his theory is wild, romantic, absurd, and dangerous; a ridiculous mixture of magic, astrology, and chemistry. (4)

But who were these authors, and just why did Paracelsus find them so unequal in their learning to the accoutrements of his footwear that their books should be consigned to the bonfire?

Both Galen and Avicenna were regarded by Paracelsus' contemporaries as twin pillars of the medical establishment and authorities in medical science and practice. They were immortalised not only by their own writings but by their many devotees who used and reused their ideas. Their stature as founding fathers of medicine was further evidenced by their inclusion alongside Hippocrates in the 14th century works of Dante and Chaucer.

In the Inferno (Canto IV 143), Dante describes how his Pilgrim is led through the First Circle of Hell, where he sees the shades of the virtuous pagans. Within the castle there he

sees 'Hippocrates, Galen, Avicenna'. (5)   Similarly, in the
General Prologue of *The Canterbury Tales* Chaucer tells us that
the Physician amongst the pilgrims was well-read in '...Ancient
Hippocrates, Hali and Galen, Avicenna, Rhazes and
Serapion...' (6)

Thus, Galen and Avicenna were regularly spoken of in the
same breath as Hippocrates, but upon what were these
reputations built?

Galen

Born into a wealthy family in Pergamon (now in modern day
Turkey) in 129 CE, Galen or Claudius Galenus grew up in the
Roman Empire at the height of its power. (7,8) (fig. 2.2) He
was originally destined to be a politician or a philosopher. His
father, however, is reported to have received instruction in a
dream from the Greek god of medicine to have his son trained
in the healing arts. At the age of 16, he began his studies in
Pergamon, which at the time was a cultural and intellectual
centre.   Three years later his father died and Galen found
himself suddenly independently wealthy. Using his new-found
resources, he decided to travel in order to expand his medical
knowledge and experience.   He visited several centres of
learning including Smyrna, Corinth and lastly Alexandria. In
157 CE at the age of 28, he returned home and was appointed
to the prestigious role of physician to the gladiators. This post
allowed him to expand further his knowledge of trauma and
human anatomy. Four years later the gladiatorial games were
suspended due to war and Galen decided to travel to Rome
where he found fame and success, eventually become the
personal physician of the imperial family. He continued to
practise, write and move in the highest tier of Roman society
until his death in around 216 CE.

Galen is thought to be the most prolific author of antiquity,
producing around 600 books, of which only around one third

survive. He wrote on diverse subjects including all aspects of medicine, anatomy and physiology as well as philology and philosophy, and any attempt to discuss his output can hardly do justice to its breadth and depth. For our current discussion, it is best to concentrate on one aspect of Galen's work — his therapeutics.

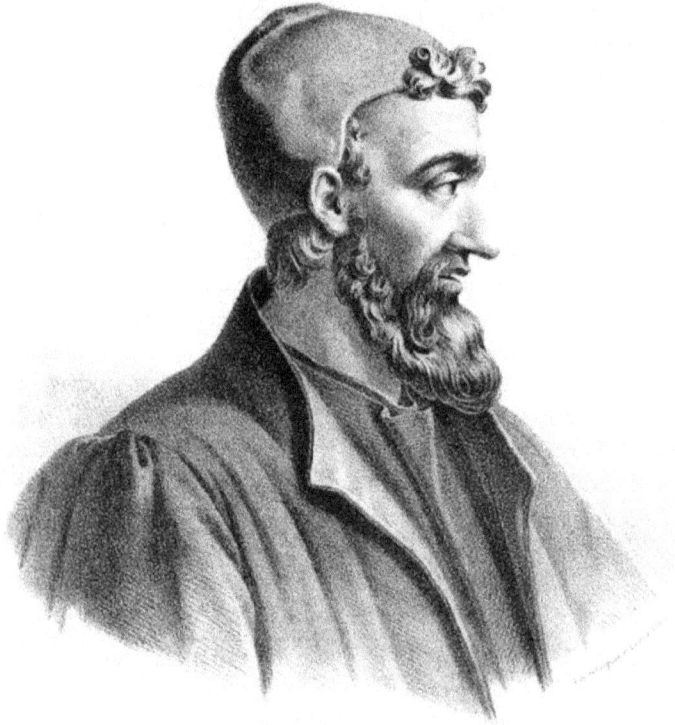

Figure 2.2. Galen of Pergamon, Lithograph by Pierre Roche Vigneron (Paris: Lithograph by Gregoire et Deneux, c1865). (CC Attribution: Andrew.Lorenzs)

Galen's treatise *On the Mixtures and Powers of Simple Drugs* was widely known and followed in both western and middle-eastern medical traditions. (9) It consists of two parts. The first part, comprising Books I-V, contains a theoretical exposition of the mechanisms of action of simple drugs, assigning them primary effective qualities (hot and cold; dry and moist), secondary qualities (e.g. relaxing, astringent, softening, hardening) and tertiary qualities (e.g. purging, diuretic, sweat-causing). The second part, comprising Books VI-XI, consists of an alphabetical listing of simple drugs and serves as a pharmacopoeia. Much of the latter half was thought to be lost, but recent work has uncovered a manuscript that may contain the missing text. At the time of writing, this is still being translated and analysed. (10)

It is the first part of Galen's treatise that distinguishes it from previous formularies, e.g. Dioscorides' famous *De Materia Medica*, as it outlines a theoretical framework for the study and practical 'use of simple medicines according to the right method'. Here, we are seeing an early attempt at systematic classification and an application of logic to the appropriate use of drugs. However, it is not merely an example of the application of reason, but also a call for experimentation.

In Book III of his treatise, Galen specifically highlights the necessity of experience in order to know and properly estimate the powers of medicines. The need for such an empirical approach is based on the realisation that, 'it is unimportant whether a substance is innately warm, cold, moist or dry; rather what is important is whether it acts warming, cooling, etc. in the human body.' (7) In other words, despite his elaborate hierarchical structure of the qualities of drugs, Galen realised that the proof of the pudding was, quite literally, in the eating.

Today, Galen is often seen as a force that held back the progress of medicine, especially because of his adherence to, and elaboration of, the Hippocratic humoral theory of disease.

In this we have the belief that all matter, including the human body, is composed of the four elements: earth, air, fire and water. In addition, the human constitution was thought to comprise the four humours or vital fluids that correspond to these elements. These were: Blood (hot and wet: element, air); Phlegm (cold and wet: element water); Black bile (melancholia) (cold and dry: element, earth); Yellow bile (choler) (hot and dry: element, fire). Disease was thought to be due to an imbalance in these humours and people's characters were also thought to be defined by them — e.g. sanguine, phlegmatic, melancholic and choleric.

However, the problem was with Galen's unquestioned authority, not with Galen himself. His thoughts on the humoral theory and even mistakes he made in his understanding of human anatomy went unchallenged for 1,400 years. But, he would have been the first to question his own beliefs. He wrote:

> I will trust no statements until I have tested them for myself as far as it has been possible for me to put them to the test. So if anyone after me becomes, like me, fond of work and zealous for truth, let him not conclude hastily from two or three cases. Often, he will be enlightened through long experience as I have. (11,12)

Although Galen placed great store in the Hippocratic writings, which were already more than 500 years old when he was studying them, he was keen not to take things at face value. Galen believed that the practice of medicine would advance through a combination of reason and experience, adding,

> The surest judge of all will be experience alone, and those who abandon it and reason on any other basis not only are deceived but destroy the value of the treatise (11,12).

28

Avicenna

Almost 800 years after Galen's death, in 980 CE, in a village near Bukhara (an ancient city on the Silk Road in present day Uzbekistan) Abu 'Ali al-Husayn ibn 'Abd Allah ibn Sina was born. (13, 14) He was a child prodigy, who is said to have memorised the Qur'an by the age of ten, and would become known as Ibn Sina, or in the West as Avicenna, one of the most celebrated Persian physician-scientists and philosophers of Islam's golden age. He died in 1037 CE, but his influence lived on through his writings. Avicenna's approach to medicine owed a great deal to the teachings of Hippocrates and Galen and indeed the perpetuation of the Hippocratic and Galenic traditions of medicine into the mediaeval world are often attributed to his writings. These writings, however, not only incorporated much of Galen's ideas, but also assimilated works from Persian, Arabian and Ayurvedic texts, as well as Avicenna's own experience.

In approximately 1012 CE, Avicenna began work on what would become his medical masterpiece, the *Kitab al-Qanun fi al-tibb* or *Canon of Medicine*. This work, consisting of five books, would be translated into Latin in the 12th century and was to become a standard European medical textbook for the next 400 years. (figs 2.3 & 2.4) Like Dioscorides' preface to his *De Materia Medica*, Avicenna in his introduction acknowledges that his work was written 'at the request of one of my very special friends, one whom I feel most bound to consider, that I prepare this book on Medicine, setting forth its general and particular laws to the full extent necessary, and yet with apt brevity.' (15)

Avicenna's opening sentences in the Canon then set out his main thesis of medicine,

> Medicine is the science by which we learn
> (a) the various states of the human body (i) in health, (ii)

29

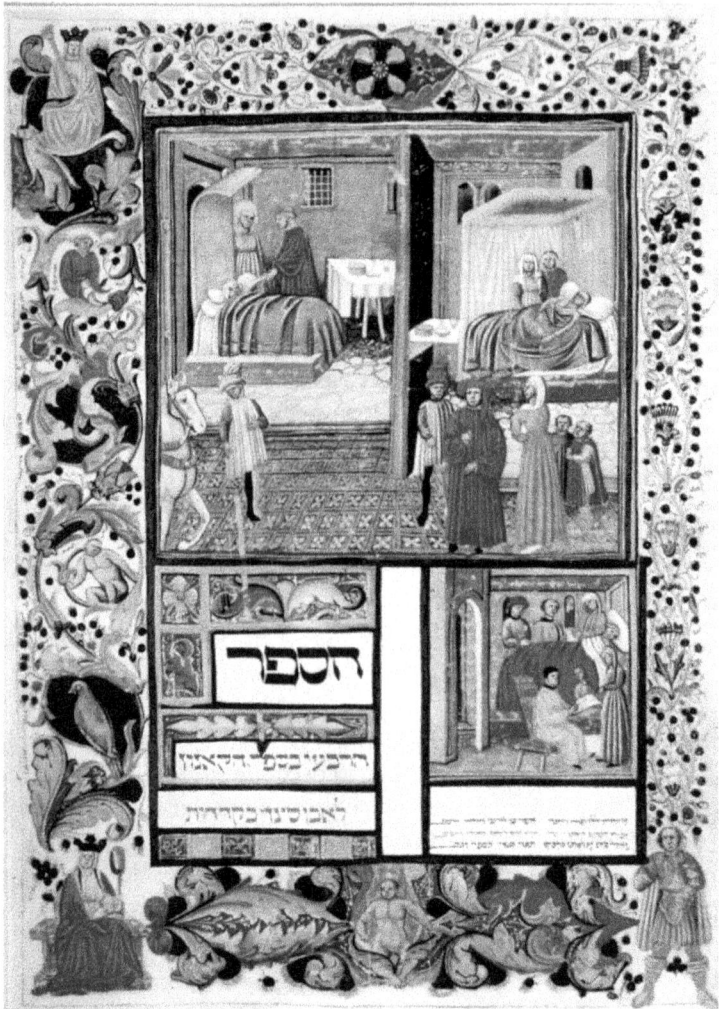

Figure 2.3. Reproduction of an illuminated page from Avicenna's Canon. Represented in the two miniatures shown here are the three basic stages of a physician's visit with a patient; the examination of the patient, the consultation with attendants, and possibly a written prescription or treatment procedure. [Courtesy of Images from the History of Medicine (NLM): Public Domain]

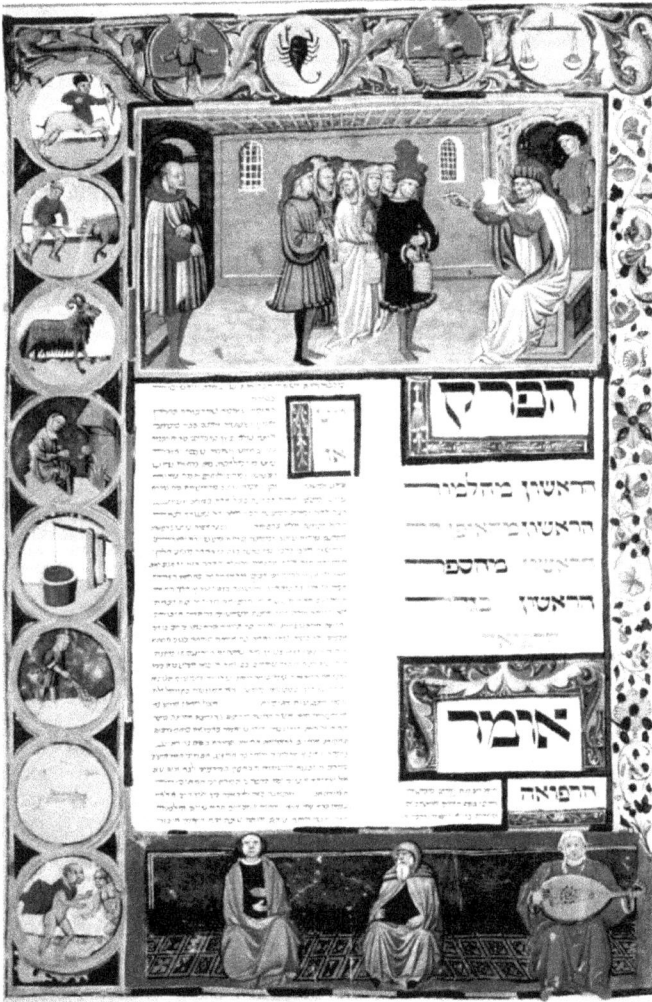

Figure 2.4. Reproduction of an illuminated page from Avicenna's Canon. This miniature shows a doctor performing urine analysis. There is a group of patients, each holding a *matula* (the vessel in which urine is collected), awaiting their turn with the doctor. The top and left borders show zodiacal figures. [Courtesy of Images from the History of Medicine (NLM): Public Domain]

when not in health,
(b) the means by which, (i) health is likely to be lost, and
(ii) when lost, is likely to be restored to health.

In other words, it is the art whereby health (the beauty
of the body — long hair, clear complexion, fragrance
and form) is conserved and the art whereby it is
restored, after being lost. (15)

Book Two of Avicenna's Canon is entitled *On Simple Drugs* or
Materia Medica. In chapter two of this book, entitled, *On
knowledge of the potency of drugs through experimentation*, he lists
seven rules that should be followed when assessing the actions
of a drug. These have recently been translated by Nasser and
colleagues (13) and here we have one of the first expositions of
a systematic and scientific approach to therapeutics.

First, Avicenna emphasises the need for purity of the drug
under scrutiny,

1. The drug must be free from any acquired quality: this
can occur if the drug is exposed to temporary heat or
cold, if there is a change in the essence of the drug, or if
the drug is in close proximity to another substance.

Next, he demonstrates his understanding of the importance of
controlled variables in any experiment,

2. The experiment must be done on a single, not a
composite, condition.

Then, he acknowledges that a drug under study may exert its
effect by curing the underlying condition or merely relieving
one its symptoms,

3. The drug must be tested on two contrary conditions.
If it is effective on both, we cannot judge which

condition benefited directly from the drug.

Despite his adherence to Galen's notion of a drug's primary effective qualities of heat and cold, dry and moist, Avicenna emphasises in his fourth rule the importance of dose escalation in the study of any new drug,

> 4. The potency of the drug should be equal to the strength of the disease... So it is best to experiment first using the weakest [dosage] and then increase it gradually until you know the potency of the drug, leaving no room for doubt.

In his next two rules, Avicenna is keen to avoid the confounding effects of chance by insisting that the timescale of any effect and its reproducibility should be studied and considered,

> 5. One should consider the time needed for the drug to take effect. If the drug has an immediate effect, this shows that it has acted against the disease itself. If its initial effect is contrary to what comes later, or if there is no initial effect at first and the effect shows up later, this leads to uncertainty and confusion. Actions in such cases could be accidental: their effect is hidden at first and later comes into the open. The confusion and uncertainty relate to the potency of the drug.

> 6. The effect of the drug should be the same in all cases or, at least, in most. If that is not the case, the effect is then accidental...

Finally, Avicenna recognises the importance of human testing and the pitfalls of relying solely on animal testing,

> 7. Experiments should be carried out on the human body. If the experiment is carried out on the bodies of

[other animals] it is possible that it might fail...

In Avicenna's rules, we have a major step forward towards the scientific method, especially as applied to therapeutics. This approach would be further developed and refined by several great minds over the ensuing centuries.

Avicenna's seven rules were taken, at least in part, from Galen who in his *De Simplicium Medicamentorum* (16) expounded on how drugs should be studied experimentally. In particular, Galen had proposed a number of principles that should be applied when testing the potency and effectiveness of drugs. These are not presented as a simple, coherent list, like Avicenna's, but are dispersed throughout his works.

For example, regarding drug dosing, Galen writes,

> The proper proportions in the mixture we shall find conjecturally before experience, scientifically after experience.

He goes on to say that the effects of drugs should be studied in three cases — the healthy individual, the slightly ailing and the really sick, and that care should taken that the drugs themselves are pure and free from any admixture of a foreign substance (11).

Importantly, Galen counselled that no cases should be counted where any error on the part of the physician, patient or bystander had been made, or where any other foreign factor had done harm. (11). He also points out some of the difficulties of medical experimentation — e.g. the extreme unlikelihood of ever being able to observe in even two cases the same combination of symptoms and circumstances. (11) And he highlighted the danger to the life of the patient from rash experimentation. (11)

Avicenna, who was very familiar with Galen's works, was no doubt heavily influenced by these principles, but he took them further, refining, expanding and ordering them in his list of seven rules. While Avicenna may have been Galen's greatest follower, others in the medieval world were aware of Galen's works as well as those of Avicenna himself. Amongst these were the mid-13th century physicians John de St Amand and Petrus Hispanus. Close contemporaries, both these men wrote influential medical treatises and both, as we shall see, also presented sets of rules or conditions for the study of drugs.

John of St Amand

John of St Amand (c1230-1303) was a French physician, cleric and academic who taught at the University of Paris and is reputed to have been the first Western academic to comment on the works of Avicenna. (11,17)

In his *Expositio in Antidotarium Nicolai,* he listed seven rules for the experimental evaluation of 'medicinal simples' (17):

1. The medicinal simple which is being tested should be pure and free from any extraneous quality...
2. Experimentation should be with a simple and not a complicated disease.
3. The simple should be tested in two contrary types of disease...
4. The virtue of the medicine should correspond to the quality of the patient.
5. Essence and accident should not be confused...
6. The experiment should be often repeated for if a medicine is tested in the cases of five men and has a heating effect upon them all, still that is not adequate proof that it will always have a heating effect...
7. The test should be on the human body and in varying states of health. Trying the medicine on a lion may not prove anything as to its effects upon a man.

John of St Amand was familiar with Avicenna's work, and his seven rules or conditions for the study of drugs are virtually identical to those of Avicenna's, both in content and order, especially given the textual variability introduced through translation, manuscript transmission and re copying over the centuries.

Petrus Hispanus

Many scholars believe Petrus Hispanus, or Peter of Spain, became Pope John XXI and that he was probably a Portuguese physician and priest (c1215-77). (18, 19) However, the works ascribed to Petrus may have in fact been written by several different authors. Whoever wrote his medical treatises cites Galen in his discussion of 'the way of experience' and 'the way of reason' and gives six conditions required for experimentation with drugs. These are similar to those of his contemporary, John of St Amand and those of Avicenna.

His six rules are found in his *Commentaries Upon the Works of Isaac* (11),

1. The medicine administered should be free from all foreign substances
2. The patient taking it should have the disease for which it is especially intended
3. It should be given alone without admixture of other medicines
4. It should be of the opposite degree to the disease
5. We should test it not once only but many times
6. The experiments should be with the proper body, as on the body of a man and not of an ass.

Petrus Hispanus' list of six rules is simpler than that of either Avicenna or John of St Amand, but there are similarities with Avicenna's, and, therefore, in turn with some of Galen's. The provenance of Petrus' rules is thus more difficult to define.

Conclusions

When Paracelsus burned the books of Galen and Avicenna it was obviously designed to be a piece of theatre consistent with his notoriously volatile personality, but it was also an attempt to turn a new page in the history of medicine. However, others before Paracelsus had already begun to write on that next page. While the middle ages are usually regarded as a dark time that would only be illuminated by the light of the renaissance, there were physicians, scientists and scholars who, despite their adherence to the authority of antiquity, could still ask important new questions.

These individuals working throughout the 12th-16th centuries, slowly eroded the impervious shell that had been built around the sanctity of ancient texts. Across the different scientific disciplines, including medicine and what would soon become pharmacology, there was a growing realization that experimentation and direct observation were the keys to understanding.

Despite Paracelsus' showy attempt to shake off the shackles of the past, perhaps it was not Galen and Avicenna who should have been torched. These Roman and Persian physicians had done everything they could to advance the practice of medicine and place it on a firmer evidence-based foundation. Admittedly, they were constrained by their adherence to the accepted wisdom passed down through the years (in Galen's case he was overly adherent to Hippocrates, and Avicenna in turn, was a slave to Galen), but they both placed high value on personal experience and experimentation. It would no doubt have astonished both Galen and Avicenna if they had learned that their works had gone unchallenged for centuries, and it would almost certainly have grieved them that medicine had, as a result, become frozen in time. They had each taken ancient traditions and developed them. In their writings, we hear not just an impersonation of their predecessors, but their own distinctive voices.

What comes next in our story, then, is the steady development of scientific thinking as it is applied to the practice of medicine. First there is the questioning of authority and the search for new answers through experimentation, and then we see the emergence of a new medicine — one built increasingly upon evidence.

By the time we reach the 18th century, we have physicians who are interested in proving that drugs work, even if they are not yet at the stage of being able to show *how* they work. In the next chapter we will look at three of that century's most famous experimenters and for the first time we will enter the world of clinical trials.

References

1.   Ball P. *The Devil's Doctor: Paracelsus and the World of Renaissance Magic and Science.* Arrow Books, London, 2007.

2.   Paracelsus, *Selected Writings*, Ed. with an introduction by Jolande Jacobi, trans. Guterman N. Pantheon, New York, 1951.

3.   Paracelsus. http://www.sciencemuseum.org.uk/broughttolife/people/paracelsus.aspx (Accessed 8 January 2016)

4.   Percival T. (1767) Essay I. The Empiric; or arguments against the use of theory and reasoning in physic. In: *Essays Medical and Experimental: The Second Edition, Revised, and Considerably Enlarged. To Which Is Added an Appendix.* 2nd Ed Cambridge University Press, Cambridge, 2014.

5.   Dante. *The Divine Comedy Volume 1: Inferno.* Trans. Musa M. Penguin Books, New York, 1984.

6.   Chaucer G. *Canterbury Tales.* Penguin Books, London, 2005.

7.   Holmes P. Galen of Pergamon A sketch of an original eclectic and integrative practitioner, and his system of medicine. *Journal of the American Herbalists Guild* 2002; Spring/Summer: 7-18.

8.   Pearsey L. Galen: a biographical sketch. http://www.ucl.ac.uk/~ucgajpd/medicina%20antiqua/bio_gal.html (Accessed 8 January 2016)

9.   Petit C. Théorie et pratique: connaissance et diffusion du traité des *Simples* de Galien au Moyen Age, in A. Ferraces Rodríguez (Ed.) IIIᵉ Seminario internacional (*Fito-zooterapia antigua y altomedieval : textos y doctrinas*), La Coruña, 21-22 Oct. 2005, La Coruña, 2009, 79-95.

10. Bhayro S, Hawley R, Kessel G, Pormann PE. The Syriac Galen Palimpsest: progress, prospects and problems. *Journal of Semitic Studies* 2013; 58: 131-148.

11. Thorndike L. *A History of Magic and Experimental Science During the First Thirteen Centuries of Our Era.* Columbia University Press, New York, 1923.

12. Coxe JR. *The Writings of Hippocrates and Galen.* Lindsay & Blakiston, Philadelphia, 1846.

13. Nasser M, Tibi A, Savage-Smith E. Ibn Sina's Canon of Medicine: 11th century rules for assessing the effects of drugs. *James Lind Library Bulletin: Commentaries on the history of treatment evaluation* 2007. http://www.jameslindlibrary.org/articles/ibn-sinas-canon-of-medicine-11th-century-rules-for-assessing-the-effects-of-drugs/ (Accessed 8 January 2016)

14. Saffari M, Pakpour AH. Avicenna's Canon of Medicine: a look at health, public health, and environmental sanitation. *Archives of Iranian Medicine* 2012; 15: 785-9.

15. Gruner OC. The *Canon of Medicine* of Avicenna (1930 English Translation of Book 1) AMS Press Inc., New York, 1973.

16. Kühn KG (Ed). *De Simplicium Medicamentorum* In: Claudii Galeni Opera Omnia, Volume 12. Cambridge University Press, Cambridge, 1821.

17. Brater DC, Daly WJ. Clinical pharmacology in the Middle Ages: principles that presage the 21st century. *Clinical Pharmacology & Therapeutics* 2000; 67: 447-50.

18. Spruyt J. Peter of Spain In: *The Stanford Encyclopedia of Philosophy* (Winter 2012 Edition), Zalta EN (Ed.) http://plato.stanford.edu/archives/win2012/entries/peter-spain/ (Accessed 8 January 2016)

19. Ambrose CT. Medicus Petrus Hispanus (c1205–77 Peter of Spain): a XIII century Pope and author of a medieval sex guide. *Journal of Medical Biography* 2013; 21: 85-94.

——— ■ ———

3

Oranges, Foxgloves and Blossom

The Beginnings of Clinical Research

Introduction

While there have been examples of clinical investigation, i.e. studies involving human participants, in our story so far, none of these can really merit the title of 'research'. This term implies a systematic approach to address scientific questions, in our case relating to the effectiveness and safety of drug treatments, and it is an essential part of modern drug development. Without well-designed, carefully conducted and expertly analysed clinical trials, no new drug today could hope to obtain the necessary authorizations for marketing and use.

It may seem that such an approach is an entirely modern one, but the origins of these rigorous strategies are once again to be found centuries ago. As we enter the 18th century, we encounter three important early examples that have for many defined the approaches we use today. The studies in question were conducted by three near contemporaries: the physicians James Lind, William Withering and Edward Jenner. They were certainly not the first ever to conduct clinical trials, nor were they the first to document them, but they have become widely regarded as the founders of modern clinical research. Largely, what they did has stood the test of time and is regarded even today as an example of rational scientific experimentation involving meticulous observation, careful analysis and the dissemination of results.

James Lind

James Lind (1716-94) (fig. 3.1) was born in Edinburgh and was initially apprenticed at the age of 15 to George Langlands, a member of the Incorporation of Surgeons, the predecessor of the Royal College of Surgeons. (1, 2) After completing eight years of training, he joined the Royal Navy as a Surgeon's Mate and for the next nine years served on board ships in the Mediterranean, West Indies and off the coast of West Africa, as well as closer to home in the English Channel. By 1747, he was now a Surgeon and serving on the *HMS Salisbury*, a brand new 50-gun ship of the line, which was patrolling the Bay of Biscay and the western approaches to the English Channel. It was while aboard the *Salisbury* that Lind turned his attentions to scurvy. (2)

From the mid-16th century, countless sailors from around the world had taken to the seas on long intercontinental voyages. Months, often years, were spent away from land, for international trade or naval warfare. For the vast majority, on-board conditions were extremely poor. The ships were over-crowded and provisions were limited by the practicalities of storing and preserving food over many months at sea. A standard sailor's diet included salt beef or pork, dried fish, hard tack or biscuit, butter, cheese, peas and beer. (1) Such a restricted diet over many months at sea led to deficiency diseases amongst the men, most notably scurvy — the consequence of vitamin C deficiency.

Scurvy was a major health problem throughout the age of sail, but historians differ in their estimates of its impact. Some claim that more than 2 million sailors perished from the ravages of this disease; a number greater than those killed by storms, shipwreck and combat combined. (1) However, others claim that diseases such as typhus may have confounded these figures. Whatever the exact numbers, it was a deadly constant and greatly feared by sailors. One account, illustrating the extent of scurvy's brutality, details Lord Anson's epic journey around the world. In 1740, while Britain was at war with Spain, he led a fleet of six warships and almost 2,000 sailors on a circumnavigation of the globe. Four years later, Anson returned with just one ship and 188 men, with reports that scurvy was responsible for 997 of the deaths. (3) Such an account was not rare. Indeed, during the Seven Years' War with France, of almost 185,000 sailors, more than 133,000 died of disease, and the majority of these were attributable to scurvy. Only 1,512 were believed killed in action. (4)

However, not all voyages resulted in such tragic losses due to scurvy. Almost 150 years before Anson's voyage around the world, there was an outbreak of scurvy as Vasco da Gama made the long voyage from Portugal to Asia. It was observed that the ill were relieved by eating citrus fruit. (5) Furthermore, in 1601 James Lancaster set off on a three-year voyage to the Spice Islands and used lemon juice to stave off scurvy aboard one of the four ships under his command. By administering 3 spoonfuls of lemon juice to the 202 sailors on board the *Red Dragon*, it was noted that he had 'cured many of his men and preserved the rest.' (1, 5)

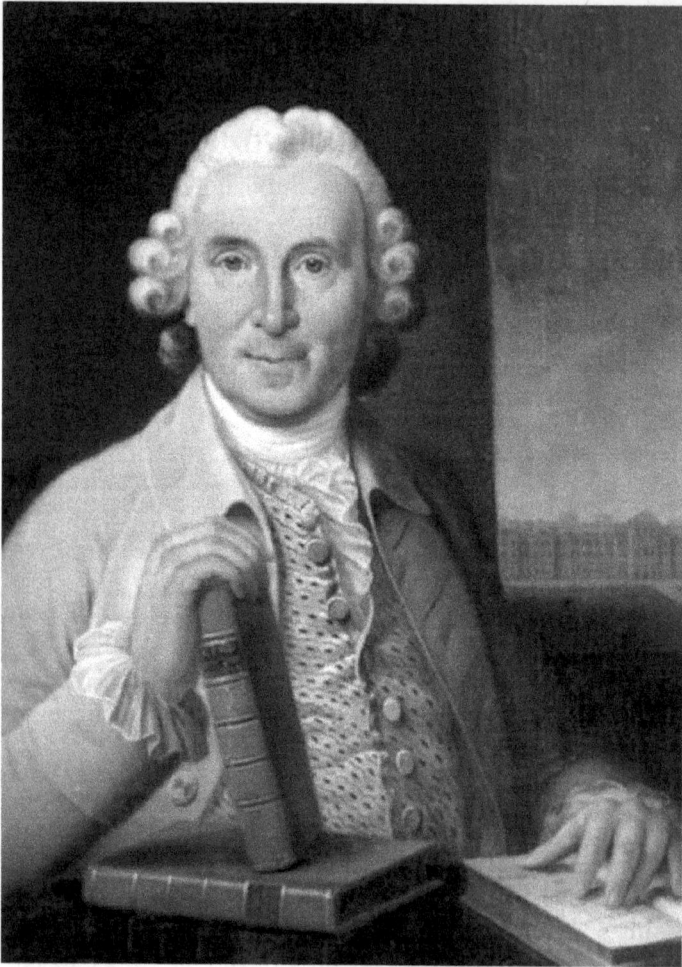

Figure 3.1. James Lind (1716-94). Detail of a painting by Sir George Chalmers c1760. (Public Domain) Lind is depicted with his *Treatise on the Scurvy* and in the background is the Navy Hospital at Haslar of which he was appointed Director in 1758.

It would appear that by the early 17th century a means to prevent and cure scurvy had already been identified by the keen observational skills of sailors. Unfortunately, the situation was greatly confused by a plethora of theories about scurvy, and its potential cures, from the eminent physicians of the day. Unlike those who advocated citrus fruits, many of the well-regarded physicians had never actually seen a man with scurvy and based the entirety of their recommendations on the prevailing medical theories of the day. Unfortunately, those who believed in the benefits of oranges and lemons could not explain their mechanism of action. Thus, despite their efficacy, the Admiralty chose instead to implement the bizarre therapies proposed by others which were, theoretically, entirely plausible in the context of 17th century medicine. Such therapies included the ingestion of sea-water, vinegar, oil of vitriol (dilute sulphuric acid) and malt wort (a sweetened soaked malt extract). (1)

With the benefits of citrus fruits practically forgotten, scurvy continued to rage through the ships during the early 18th century. Many therapies were recommended without proof of their efficacy until Lind attempted to clarify the situation. He was acutely aware of the impact of scurvy and the urgency with which a solution was required, when he said:

> the scurvy alone, during the last war, proved a more destructive enemy, and cut off more valuable lives, than the united efforts of the French and Spanish arms. (6)

Thus, six weeks after leaving port, on the last of six patrols of the Channel, Lind conducted what has since become his world famous clinical trial.

> On the 20th of May, 1747, I took twelve patients in the scurvy, on board the Salisbury at sea. Their cases were as similar as I could have them. They all in general had putrid gums, the spots and lassitude, with weakness of their knees. ... and had one diet common to all... Two

of these were ordered each a quart of cyder a-day. Two others took twenty-five gutts of elixir vitriol three times a-day.... Two others took two spoonfuls of vinegar three times a-day...; Two of the worst patients...were put under a course of sea-water... Two others had each two oranges and one lemon given them every day. These they ate with greediness, at different times, upon an empty stomach. They continued but six days under this course, having consumed the quantity that could be spared. The two remaining patients, took the bigness of a nutmeg three times a-day.... The consequence was, that the most sudden and visible good effects were perceived from the use of oranges and lemons; one of those who had taken them, being at the end of six days fit for duty.... The other was the best recovered of any in his condition; and being now deemed pretty well, was appointed nurse to the rest of the sick. (6)

His results were conclusive. By using a set of carefully conducted, controlled clinical experiments Lind was able to demonstrate that those who ate citrus fruits recovered, while those who took other standard therapies of the time did not. His experiments clarified the situation and seemed to address the confusion caused by the many unfounded recommendations, which hampered the management of scurvy.

In 1748, Lind left the Navy. He returned to Edinburgh where he completed his MD thesis in venereal disease, another scourge of the Navy, and began working as a physician. Five years later, he published the findings of his experiments in his *Treatise on The Scurvy, Containing an Inquiry into the Nature, Causes, and Cure, of that Disease Together with A Critical and Chronological View on what has been Published on the Subject.* (fig. 3.2) (6)

Importantly, in his book, Lind first undertook a review of the literature. By critically appraising previously published works he attempted to address the deficiencies in the many theories, which acted as barriers to the effective treatment of scurvy. He recognised that 'Indeed, before this subject could be set in a clear and proper light, it was necessary to remove a great deal of rubbish' but insisted,

> where I have been necessarily led, in this disagreeable part of the work, to criticise the sentiments of eminent and learned authors, I have not done it with a malignant view of depreciating their labours, or their names; but from a regard to truth, and the good of mankind. (6)

He published the findings of his experiments and offered his conclusions in 1753. However, despite correctly identifying citrus fruits as a cure for scurvy, it was not until 1795 — the year after Lind's death — that the Admiralty began the routine issue of lemon juice to their sailors for the prevention of scurvy.

It may seem incongruous that a cure for a serious and highly prevalent disease should be conclusively demonstrated, yet not implemented for over 40 years. However, there are a number of possible reasons.

In Lind's case, personal and professional credibility may have contributed to his failure to convince the Admiralty to adopt his method of preventing scurvy as routine practice. Although the publication of his *Treatise on The Scurvy* made his reputation and allowed his appointment as director of the new Navy Hospital at Haslar in 1758, unlike his contemporaries, he began life in the Navy as a lowly Surgeon's Mate, having come from a family without influential connections. Perhaps, had he a higher social standing it may not have taken 42 years for the recommendations of his *Treatise* to be implemented. For example, Gilbert Blane, a Scottish physician from an upper class family, Physician to the Fleet and later Commissioner on the Board of the Sick and Wounded Sailors, was subsequently instrumental in the introduction of daily rationing of lemon juice for all sailors in 1795.

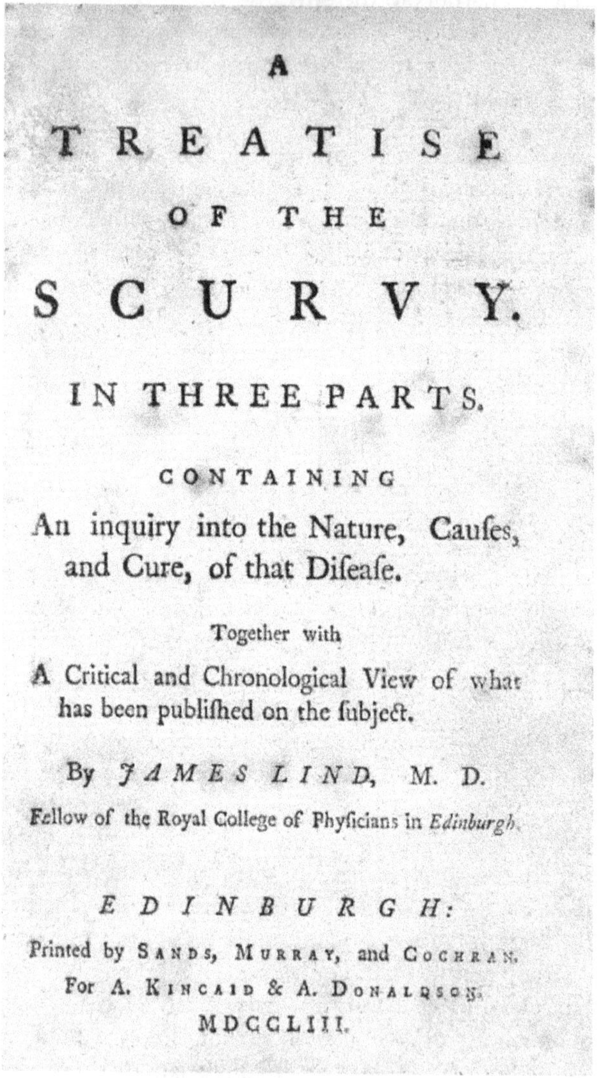

A

TREATISE

OF THE

SCURVY.

IN THREE PARTS.

CONTAINING

An inquiry into the Nature, Causes, and Cure, of that Disease.

Together with

A Critical and Chronological View of what has been published on the subject.

By *JAMES LIND*, M. D.

Fellow of the Royal College of Physicians in *Edinburgh*.

EDINBURGH:

Printed by SANDS, MURRAY, and COCHRAN.
For A. KINCAID & A. DONALDSON.
MDCCLIII.

Figure 3.2. Frontispiece of the first edition of Lind's Treatise on the Scurvy, published in 1753.

However, there were a number of other reasons that contributed to this delay. Although Lind demonstrated that oranges and lemons were effective in curing scurvy, he did not appreciate that a lack of one of their key constituents was its cause, nor their mechanism of action. Lind believed that the acids of oranges and lemons had some special quality, and hence their efficacy over vinegar and oil of vitriol, which were standard therapies at the time.

He also recognised that the practicalities of transporting enough fresh fruit for many hundreds of sailors on long voyages lacked feasibility. He therefore recommended a method by which the 'virtues of twelve dozen lemons or oranges, may be put into a quart-bottle and preserved for years.' (1) His proposed method involved concentrating lemon juice into a 'rob' by heating it and unknowingly depleting its vitamin C content. Although some vitamin C would have been preserved in the 'rob', it was a concentrate and given in small doses, meaning that it was ineffective. The 'rob' was expensive to produce and given its inert nature, it was perhaps unsurprising that this recommendation failed to be adopted aboard Navy vessels.

What was surprising, however, was that having undertaken his previous study with such scientific rigour, Lind proposed his 'rob' without evidence of its efficacy — an approach he had derided others for in his literature review on scurvy. Had he been consistent in his methodology, he might have developed an understanding of the mechanism of action of citrus fruits, and been able to make a more informed recommendation.

Finally, not only did Lind hail from a humble background but also, by strongly criticising the theories and treatments of the most eminent physicians of the day, he may have alienated them. Thus, his own recommendations may not have received the support they would have needed from the very physicians he openly attacked.

William Withering

While Lind was serving at sea as a Surgeon's Mate, William Withering (1741-99) was born in Shropshire. (fig. 3.3) Like Lind, he spent some time apprenticed to a local surgeon, but in 1762, at the age of 21, he went to Edinburgh University to study medicine. (7, 8) In his final year, 1765/66, he submitted his thesis on *Malignant Putrid Sore Throat*, which earned him his MD.

In 1766, he travelled to France and as part of his medical education visited one of the oldest hospitals in the world — the famous Hôtel Dieu in Paris. On his return, he set up practice in Stafford, but soon moved to take a more financially secure position as a hospital physician in Birmingham General in 1775. (7) He was a successful physician, so much so that he is reputed to have had the largest practice outside of London. But, despite his extensive medical work he adopted the philosophy of the Enlightenment, that an educated man should endeavour to learn all that it was possible to know. Correspondingly, his interests and his work crossed a range of disciplines.

He was first a celebrated botanist, despite eschewing the study while a medical student at university, and he published an important book on the subject in 1776, *The Botanical Arrangement of all Vegetables Naturally Growing in Great Britain* (9), which in various editions would be in print for the next century. In this work, he adopted a rigorous approach using the Linnaean system of nomenclature and he was clear in his thoughts for the need for an empirical approach when he wrote,

> we shall sooner obtain the end proposed if we take up the subject as altogether new and, rejecting the fables of the ancient herbalist, build only upon the basis of accurate and well considered experiments. (9)

This was very much the strategy he adopted when later he would combine his interests in botany and medicine in his drug research. He was also a geologist and indeed his election as a Fellow of the Royal Society was on the basis of this pursuit. Withering had both a plant and a mineral named in his honour during his lifetime, but what he is best remembered for today is his work on the foxglove.

Preparations of the wildflower purple foxglove (*Digitalis purpurea*) had been used since antiquity for the treatment of dropsy or water retention, most commonly due to congestive cardiac failure. The foxglove as a therapeutic plant is mentioned by both Dioscorides and Galen, and the 16th century German physician and botanist Leonard Fuchs named the plant *Digitalis* and recommended it for the 'scattering of dropsy'. Withering would have been acquainted with these precedents and was well primed when he was asked about a secret family recipe for dropsy kept by 'an old woman in Shropshire, who had sometimes made cures after the more regular practitioners had failed.' (10, 11)

He noted that her herbal remedy, 'was composed of twenty or more different herbs; but it was not very difficult for one conversant in these subjects, to perceive, that the active herb could be no other than the Foxglove.'(10) And, he concluded, 'the Digitalis purpurea merited more attention than modern practice bestowed upon it.' (9)

Withering was aware of much anecdotal evidence for the effectiveness of foxglove preparations, but he was equally aware of the many reports of its significant toxicity. There were many unknowns about its use. Which part of the plant was active, in which season should it be gathered, how should it be prepared and perhaps most importantly, what dose should be administered and for how long?

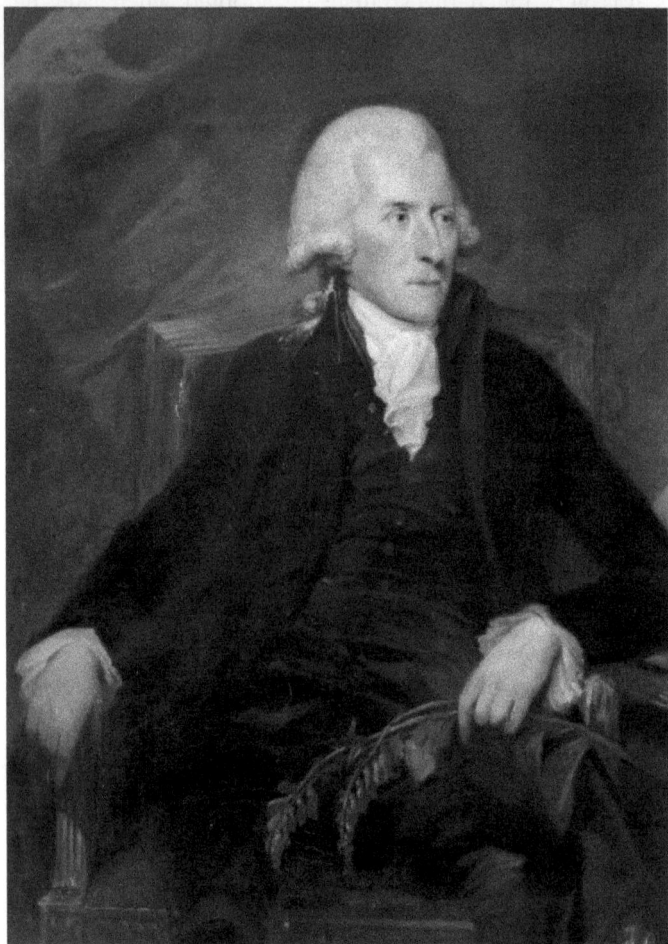

Figure 3.3. William Withering (1741-99), after a painting by Carl Frederik von Breda (With Permission of the University of Birmingham, UK). Withering is depicted holding the purple foxglove.

He established that the dried leaves of the plant were significantly more effective than fresh ones and that powdered, dried leaves were better than any decoction, or extraction made by boiling. Although unknown to Withering, the latter process would have destroyed the active component.

In his published account of 1785, he reports on 163 patients treated over a nine-year period and also includes a large number of case studies submitted to him by other physicians. (10) (fig. 3.4) From these studies he made a number of important conclusions.

First, he found that many physicians, including himself, had been using excessive doses of the drug and that this had contributed to the observed toxicity. In relation to this, he characterized the principal adverse effects of digitalis as nausea, vomiting, diarrhoea and visual disturbances with 'objects appearing green or yellow'. The onset of such toxic side-effects, Withering concluded, should prompt the physician to stop the treatment.

He also found that not all his cases of dropsy responded. Digitalis is a cardiac glycoside having its primary action on the heart muscle, where it effectively increases the strength of contraction and affects cardiac rhythm. As such, those cases of dropsy resulting from congestive cardiac failure would respond and others, such as those due to liver cirrhosis, would not. Approximately 100 of Withering's cases are consistent with a cardiac diagnosis and the majority of those were treated effectively with digitalis. The other cases were likely due to a range of other causes and many of these were unrelieved by treatment. Although the mechanism of action would take another century to unravel (12), Withering was aware that his digitalis preparations were having cardiac effects.

Withering was also aware of the problem of anecdotal reporting that was so prevalent in his time, and he counseled caution against what we would now call 'reporting bias' (13) when he wrote,

> It would have been an easy task to have given select cases, whose successful treatment would have spoken strongly in favour of the medicine, and perhaps been flattering to my own reputation. But Truth and Science would condemn the procedure. I have therefore mentioned every case... proper or improper, successful or otherwise. (10)

Despite these findings, Withering was well aware of the need for further research in order to fully understand the medical use of digitalis, and he concludes the preface of his book with the words,

> After all, in spite of opinion, prejudice, or error, Time will fix the real value upon this discovery, and determine whether I have imposed upon myself and others, or contributed to the benefit of science and mankind. (10)

Time has passed, and digitalis and its close relative digoxin are still used in modern medical practice. The side effect profile we see with overdosage is as Withering described it, and the basic principles of treatment are as he defined them. His work, performed over 200 years ago stands the test of time and has, in the intervening centuries provided relief to countless patients.

AN

A C C O U N T

OF THE

FOXGLOVE,

AND

Some of its Medical Ufes :

WITH

PRACTICAL REMARKS ON DROPSY,

AND OTHER DISEASES.

BY

WILLIAM WITHERING, M. D.

Phyfician to the General Hofpital at Birmingham.

—— nonumque prematur in annum.

HORACE.

BIRMINGHAM: PRINTED BY M. SWINNEY;

FOR

G. G. J. AND J. ROBINSON, PATERNOSTER-ROW, LONDON

M,DCC,LXXXV.

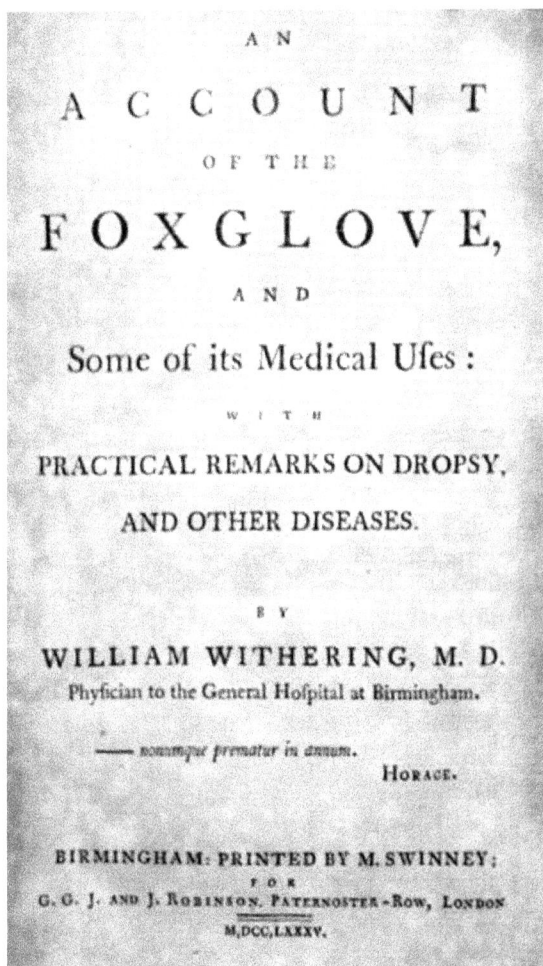

Figure 3.4. Frontispiece of Withering's work on the foxglove. The Latin inscription '*nonumque prematur in annum*' is a quotation from Horace's *Art of Poetry* and translates approximately as, 'Let it (your first draft) be held back from publication until the ninth year' and is doubtless an allusion to the nine years of case studies Withering presents in the book.

55

Edward Jenner

Two years after Lind performed his clinical trial and while Withering was in elementary school, Edward Jenner (1749-1823) was born in Berkeley, Gloucestershire. Like Lind and Withering, as a teenager he was apprenticed to a surgeon, with whom he worked from the age of 13 to 21. (14-16) (fig. 3.5) He then moved to London to complete his medical training under the charismatic and influential John Hunter at St. George's Medical School. At the age of 23, the same age that Lind joined the Navy, Jenner returned to his birthplace to set up practice, where he would remain for most of the rest of his life.

Like Withering, he was man of the Enlightenment and pursued diverse interests. He was a musician, a poet, a balloonist, a geologist and his interest in ornithology earned him his Fellowship of the Royal Society when he worked out that it was the cuckoo hatchling that evicted the eggs and chicks from its foster parents' nest and not the adult bird. This observation was for many years disputed, but Jenner was vindicated when, in 1921, photographic evidence supporting his conclusions was filmed. But, it is not for the study of the cuckoo that we best remember Jenner today; it is his contribution to the field of vaccination.

Smallpox is a viral disease that has had devastating effects on humans throughout history. It is associated with a high death rate — particularly in infants — and many survivors are left blind or with disfiguring scars. (16) However, it was well known throughout the ages that survivors of smallpox were immune to re-infection. It was perhaps a small logical step to think of deliberately infecting non-immune individuals with a mild case of smallpox in order to render them immune to a more serious and potentially life-threatening one.

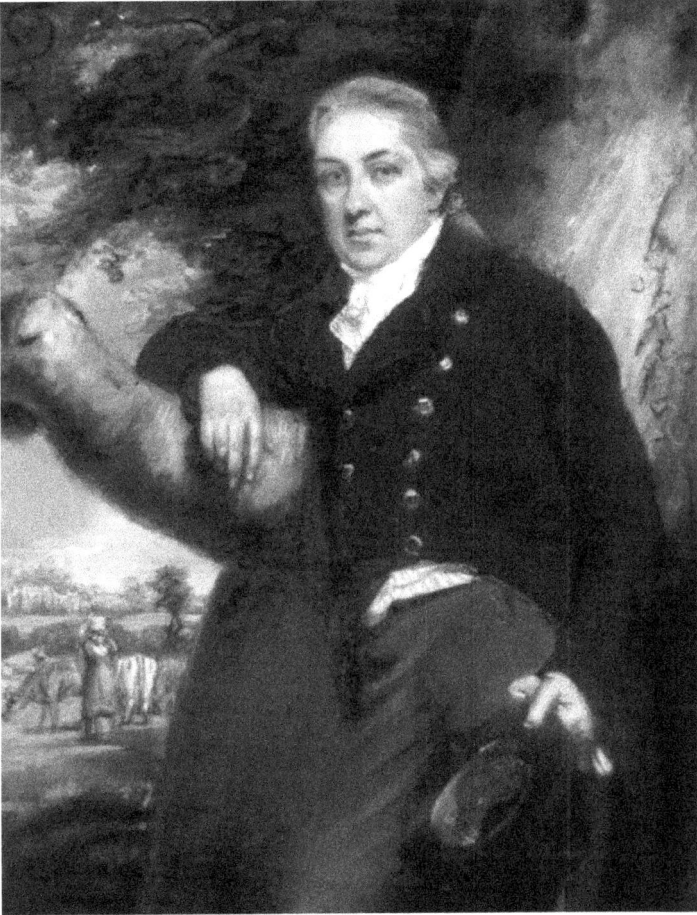

Figure 3.5. Edward Jenner (1749-1823), detail of a painting by John Raphael Smith c1800. (Public Domain) Jenner is depicted in a rural setting with a milkmaid and cows in the background.

Such a practice had been carried out since at least the 17th century and probably much longer before, and included the inoculation, or grafting, of pus from smallpox lesions under the skin of non-immune subjects. This form of inoculation was also known as *variolation* from the Latin for smallpox: *variola*. Edward Jenner himself had been variolated as an eight-year old boy, as had countless others in the first half of the 18th century. Variolation was of course potentially dangerous — not only did 2-3% of those inoculated in this way die from smallpox as a direct result of the deliberate infection, others contracted blood borne disease such as syphilis from the procedure. However, its widespread use did significantly reduce the death toll from natural infection.

The notion that the much milder infection cowpox, which milkmaids and farmers might contract from their infected cows, could protect against its more deadly viral relative, smallpox, was also widely known. (17, 18) The usual version of how Jenner came to be acquainted with this idea is that, while a surgical apprentice, he heard a dairymaid say, 'I shall never have smallpox for I have had cowpox. I shall never have an ugly pockmarked face.' (14) However, it was not only milkmaids who were aware of the protective effects of a cowpox infection; the medical profession were also well-acquainted with this form of prophylaxis. Indeed, in 1765, when the teenage Jenner was still a surgeon's apprentice, the Gloucestershire surgeon-apothecary John Frewster presented a paper to the London Medical Society entitled, *Cowpox and its ability to prevent smallpox*. Frewster also recalled discussing his findings at a local medical society dinner attended by the surgeon Daniel Ludlow and his young apprentice, Edward Jenner. (16)

Jenner then was undoubtedly aware of Frewster's work, but he may have been ignorant of that of the Dorset farmer Benjamin Jesty. (19) Jesty was as aware as any dairy farmer of the link between cowpox and immunity from smallpox. This was undoubtedly reinforced when two of his milkmaids, Anne

Notly and Mary Reade nursed their smallpox-infected relatives without contracting the disease themselves. When a smallpox outbreak threatened his own family, Jesty decided to put his observations into practice. Rather than having his wife and two toddler sons variolated, he took the bold step of inoculating them himself with cowpox. All three survived the smallpox outbreak, but Jesty was vilified locally for what he had done to his family and they moved away. This was in 1774 — some 22 years before Jenner's experiments. Intriguingly, Jesty, not a professional scientist, but clearly with a good scientific mind, tested his work by later having his sons variolated. They showed no reaction to the smallpox inoculation confirming their immunity.

It was not until the spring of 1796 that Jenner performed his first experiments. A local milkmaid called Sarah Nelms had contracted cowpox and Jenner found her to have fresh lesions on her hands. The responsible cow was called *Blossom*, whose hide and horns can be seen today in St George's Medical School and The Edward Jenner Museum respectively. There are, however, a number of other antique cow horns around that purport to be Blossom's, and unless she was a very unusual cow we might conclude that not all are authentic.

On 14 May 1796, Jenner took pus from Nelms' lesions, and inoculated the son of his gardener. The boy, James Phipps, was 8-years old at the time, and he subsequently developed a mild fever and discomfort in the axillae, but apart from these minor symptoms quickly recovered. Almost seven weeks after the cowpox inoculation, Jenner inoculated the boy again, this time with pus from a fresh smallpox lesion. Phipps, despite this challenge, did not develop the disease and Jenner concluded that he was immune.

Jenner wrote jubilantly to his friend Edward Gardner on 19 July,

As I promised to let you know how I proceeded in my

59

Inquiry into that singular disease the cowpox...I have at last accomplished what I have been so long waiting for, the passing of the vaccine Virus from one human being to another by the ordinary mode of Inoculation...I was astonished at the close resemblance of the Pustules in some of their stages to variolated Pustules. But now listen to the most delightful part of my story. The Boy has since been inoculated for the small pox which as I ventured to predict produced no effect. I shall now pursue my Experiments with redoubled ardour. (Quoted in 16)

However, first he decided to publish his experiment on Phipps and he submitted a paper to the *Philosophical Transactions* of the Royal Society, which was quickly rejected as being too premature. It took Jenner another year to get over his initial excitement and subsequent disappointment and to apply that 'redoubled ardour' to further experiments. These included identifying further human cases of cowpox and variolating them to test for immunity to smallpox, and inoculating another dozen subjects with cowpox. These were mostly children and included his own one-year old son. Jenner now felt he had enough to publish and prepared a report, which, rather than going back to the Royal Society, he chose to publish at his own expense.

An Enquiry into the causes and effects of the Variolae Vaccinae: a disease discovered in some of the Western Counties of England, particularly Gloucestershire, and known by the name of the Cow Pox was published on 17 September 1798 and despite its deficiencies — it was far from a clear, well-written, scientific report — it made Jenner famous. (20) (fig. 3.6)

The process of cowpox inoculation was soon after termed *vaccination* (from the Latin *vaccinus*, of cows) by Plymouth surgeon, Richard Dunning and almost 80 years later, Louis Pasteur proposed that all immunisations for infections should be termed vaccinations in honour of Jenner. (16)

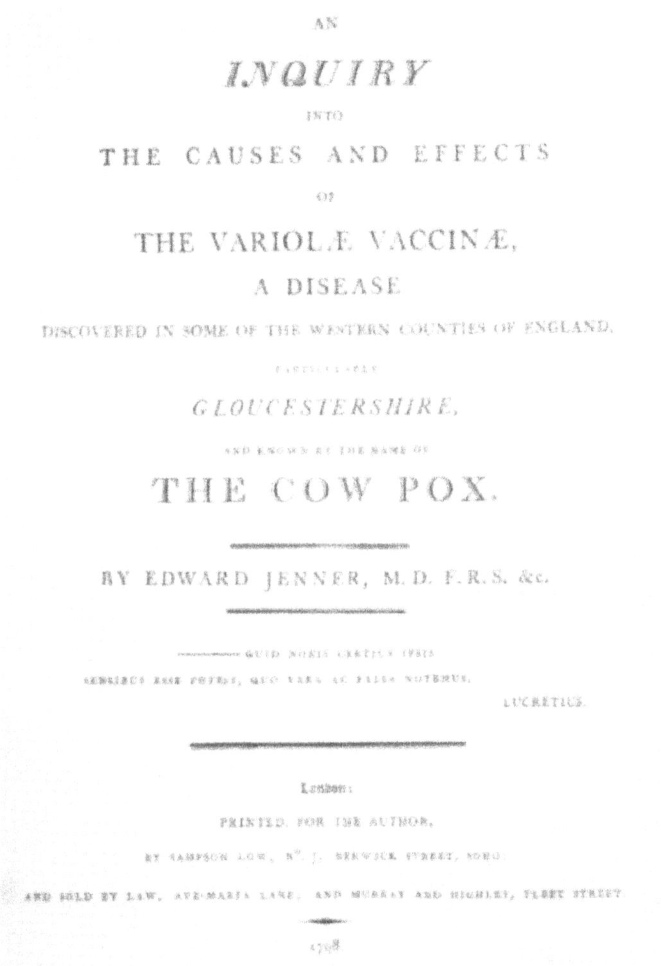

AN

I N Q U I R Y

INTO

THE CAUSES AND EFFECTS

OF

THE VARIOLÆ VACCINÆ,

A DISEASE

DISCOVERED IN SOME OF THE WESTERN COUNTIES OF ENGLAND,

PARTICULARLY

GLOUCESTERSHIRE,

AND KNOWN BY THE NAME OF

THE COW POX.

BY EDWARD JENNER, M. D. F.R.S. &c.

——— QUID NOBIS CERTIUS IPSIS
SENSIBUS ESSE POTEST, QUO VERA AC FALSA NOTEMUS.

LUCRETIUS.

London:

PRINTED FOR THE AUTHOR,

BY SAMPSON LOW, N°. 7. BERWICK STREET, SOHO:

AND SOLD BY LAW, AVE-MARIA LANE, AND MURRAY AND HIGHLEY, FLEET STREET.

1798

Figure 3.6. Frontispiece of Jenner's work *The Cow Pox*. The Latin inscription 'quid nobis certius ipsis sensibus esse potest, quo vera ac falsa notemus' is a quotation from Lucretius' *De Rerum Natura* and translates as, 'What can give us more sure knowledge than our senses? How else can we distinguish between the true and the false?'

In the years following his publication, Jenner tirelessly promoted vaccination as a preventive measure and although he was honoured in some quarters, he received nothing but ridicule in others. Undoubtedly, professional jealously played a part in the latter and after a decade Jenner decided to withdraw from the public debate and return to his roots in rural Gloucestershire, where he continued his medical practice and died in 1823. His first vaccinee, the boy Phipps, was now a married man and served as one of Jenner's pallbearers at his funeral.

What began in a country doctor's home with the inoculation of a young boy would end 184 years later when in 1980 it was declared that, following a global immunization campaign led by the WHO, smallpox had been eradicated from the world. (21)

Conclusions

Lind was not the first to proposed citrus fruit as a cure for scurvy. Withering was not the first to recognize the foxglove as a remedy for dropsy. And Jenner, was not the first to suggest, nor the first to try out inoculation with cowpox as a prevention for smallpox. Why then do we celebrate these three 18th century physicians as innovators?

There are probably several answers to that question. Without doubt, all three were highly astute observers. They each had the ability to see a problem, define its parameters and devise an experimental approach to provide an answer. More specifically, Lind understood the importance of controls, Withering the importance of reporting bias and Jenner the importance of reproducibility. In addition, all recognized the importance of publishing and disseminating their results and each also worked hard beyond their initial 'discovery' to promote its implementation in clinical practice.

Alternatively, we may choose to remember and honour these three men because it is easier to focus our attentions, however erroneously, on a single investigator rather than the disconnected teams who have really contributed. Even in science, we still perpetuate the myth of the lone genius making a medical breakthrough.

From the perspective of the present we can, however, evaluate the contributions of Lind, Withering and Jenner a little more objectively. What they each managed was to take what had previously been little more than folklore and anecdote and, through careful experimentation, place it on a firm scientific footing, and finally they told the world about it. As such their work serves as a model for what is to come.

References

1.   Bown, S. *Scurvy: How a Surgeon, a Mariner and a Gentleman Solved the Greatest Medical Mystery of the Age of the Sail.* Summersdale, Chichester, 2003.

2.   Dunn PM. James Lind (1716-94) of Edinburgh and the treatment of scurvy. *Archives of Disease in Childhood* 1997; 76: F64–5.

3.   Watt J. The medical bequest of disaster at sea: Commodore Anson's circumnavigation 1740–44. *Journal of the Royal College of Physicians London* 1998; 32: 572–9.

4.   Northcote W. *The Diseases Incident to Armies, with the Method of Cure, Translated from the Original of Baron Van Swieten, to Which Are Added the Nature and Treatment of Gun-shot Wounds, by John Ranby. Likewise Some Brief Directions to be Followed by Sea Surgeons in Engagements. Also preventatives of the scurvy at sea. Published for the use of military, and naval surgeons in America.* Philadelphia, PA: R Bell, 1776: 167.

5.   Baron JH. Sailors' scurvy before and after James Lind – a reassessment. *Nutrition Reviews* 2009; 67: 315-32.

6.   Lind J. *A Treatise of the Scurvy in Three Parts. Containing an Inquiry into the Nature, Causes and Cure of that Disease, together with a Critical and Chronological View of what has been published on the subject.* A Miller, Edinburgh, 1753.

7.   Lee MR. William Withering (1741-1799): a Birmingham Lunatic. *Proceedings of the Royal College of Physicians of Edinburgh* 2001; 31: 77-83.

8.   Norman JM. William Withering and the purple foxglove: A bicentennial tribute. *Journal of Clinical Pharmacology* 1985; 25: 479-83.

9.   Withering W. *A Botanical arrangement of all the Vegetables naturally growing in Great Britain.* London. M Winney for T Cadell, P Elmsley and G Robinson, London, 1776.

10. Withering W. *An Account of the Foxglove and Some of Its Medical Uses: With Practical Remarks on Dropsy and Other Diseases.* M. Sweeny, Birmingham, 1785.

11. Estes JW, White PD. William Withering and the purple foxglove. *Scientific American* 1965; 212: 110-9.

12. Schmiedeberg JEO: Untersuchungen ueber die pharmakologische wirksamen Bestandtheile der Digitalis purpurea. *Archiv für experimentelle Pathologie und Pharmakologie* 1875; 3: 16-43.

13. Tröhler U. Withering's 1785 appeal for caution when reporting on a new medicine. *James Lind Library Bulletin: Commentaries on the history of treatment evaluation* 2003. http://www.jameslindlibrary.org/articles/witherings-1785-appeal-for-caution-when-reporting-on-a-new-medicine/ (Accessed 8 January 2016).

14. Riedel S. Edward Jenner and the history of smallpox and vaccination. *Proceedings of Baylor University Medical Center* 2005; 18: 21-5.

15. Lakhani S. Early clinical pathologists: Edward Jenner (1749-

1823). *Journal of Clinical Pathology* 1992; 45: 756–8.

16. Williams G. *Angel of Death. The Story of Smallpox.* Palgrave Macmillan, Basingstoke, 2010.

17. Gross CP, Sepkowitz KA. The myth of the medical breakthrough: smallpox, vaccination, and Jenner reconsidered. *International Journal of Infectious Disease* 1998; 3: 54-60.

18. Mullin D. Prometheus in Gloucestershire: Edward Jenner, 1749-1823. *Journal of Allergy and Clinical Immunology* 2003; 112: 810-4.

19. Jesty R, Williams G. Who invented vaccination? *Malta Medical Journal* 2011; 23: 29-32.

20. Jenner E. *An Enquiry into the causes and effects of the Variolae Vaccinae: a disease discovered in some of the Western Counties of England, particularly Gloucestershire, and known by the name of the Cow Pox.* Sampson Low, London, 1798.

21. Global Commission for Certification of Smallpox Eradication. World Health Organization. *The Global Eradication of Smallpox: Final Report of the Global Commission for the Certification of Smallpox Eradication.* World Health Organization, Geneva, 1980.

— ■ —

4

A Search for Mechanism

The Beginnings of Pharmacology

Introduction

Like searching for the source of the Nile, unraveling the origins of an academic discipline is fraught with difficulties and uncertainty. When it comes to pharmacology, the study of drugs, or more specifically the science of drug action, there are many tributaries to navigate. Quite apart from the fact that many ancients had professional as well as personal interests in drug action, countless chemists and physiologists in more recent centuries had been regularly performing what today may be regarded as pharmacological studies. So, where does the science of pharmacology begin?

Finding a name

In the second half of the 18th century, medical practice was in turmoil after a period of relative stagnation lasting more than 500 years. Through numerous discoveries and a wholly different approach to the subject, medieval medicine was giving way to a more enlightened system. (1) As part of this, there was a growing desire to place medical practice on a much more solid scientific foundation.

The term *pharmacology* itself was probably coined in the late 17th century, but acquired its modern definition in 1791 from Friedrich Albrecht Karl Gren, a German chemist and physician. (2) He distinguished the science of the action of drugs from the mere description and collection of drugs. This cataloguing of drugs was materia medica, while pharmacology was a science. A science, however, needed a rational framework and a method. These were initially offered by the physician and philosopher Johann Christian Reil (1759-1813). (3) (fig. 4.1)

Finding a framework

Reil taught at the University of Halle for 22 years, during which time he established a high reputation as a physician, scientist and educator. During his tenure, he promoted the idea that medical practice should be grounded in physiology, which in turn should have chemistry as its foundation. Indeed, as he viewed physicians primarily as scientists, he argued that an appropriate medical education was one built on the basic sciences. (4)

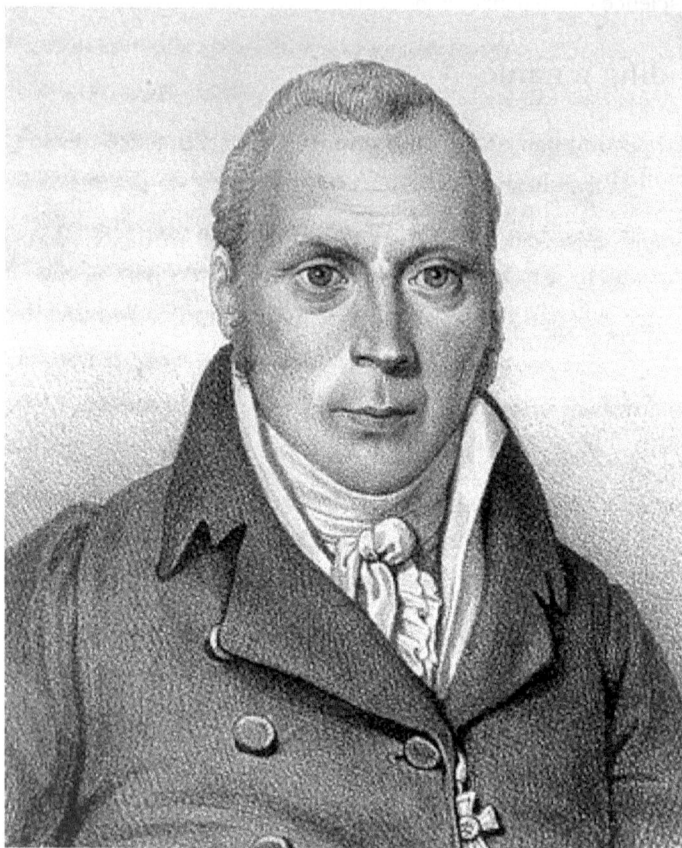

Figure 4.1. Johann Christian Reil (1759-1813) c1811. Engraving by de Frey after Leon Noel. (Wellcome Library, London)

Like many of his contemporaries, Reil had wide inter-disciplinary interests. He is remembered today primarily because of his work on the brain. In his last years at Halle, between 1807-9, he published his studies of neuroanatomy and expanded on his previous work in mental health. There are now three structures in the brain that bear his eponym: the *Island of Reil* or insula; the *Fillet of Reil*, a portion of the lateral lemniscus; and *Reil's Triangle* or the lemniscal trigone, a triangular area on the surface of the mesencephalon. (5) Reil was also especially interested in the medical treatment of those with mental illnesses. Indeed, in 1808, he first used the term *Psychiaterie* to emphasise that the management of mental illness was a core medical remit and that physicians rather than other professional groups should lead in the treatment of the mentally ill. He saw his new 'psychiatry' as inseparable from medicine and argued that Universities should issue three medical degrees: Doctorates of Surgery, Pharmacy and Psychiatry. (6)

In addition to these legacies, it was Reil's interest in therapeutics that left a lasting, if less acknowledged contribution to the developing science of pharmacology.

In 1799, he published his *Beitrag zu den Prinzipien für jede künftige Pharmakologie* (Contribution to the Principles of a Future Pharmacology), in which, like Galen, Avicenna and others before him, Reil proposed and enumerated a set of rules for the conduct of pharmacological research. (7) These were presented as a theoretical framework on which to build a scientific approach to the study and evaluation of drugs.

It is possible that Reil was aware of the published findings of James Lind (1753), William Withering (1785) and Edward Jenner (1798) all of whom had exemplified at least some of the principles he proposed. He may also have been familiar with the work of Avicenna who, as we have seen in chapter 2, almost 800 years earlier had proposed a similar set of rules for the study and evaluation of new drugs.

Reil begins his treatise with his definition of the subject. 'Pharmacology' he notes, 'should explain the effects of certain substances, i.e. drugs, on the human body.' (7) He goes on to expand upon this when he asks, 'What does pharmacology have to offer?' He answers his own question: 'it has to explain factually and scientifically to the last detail those changes that arise in the interaction between a medical substance and a living being. The drug may also undergo changes which interest us only insofar as they contribute to the explanation of the changes to the human body.' Here, Reil puts forward the notion that not only do drugs affect the body, but that the body also affects drugs, thus presciently proposing the idea of drug metabolism long before such a concept would be confirmed.

To understand this interaction of drug and living system, Reil goes on to say that we need,

> A complete understanding of every aspect of the nature of drugs, especially with regard to their chemical makeup..., a complete understanding of the physical nature of the human being, the basic combination of his various organs, his strengths, the combination of the organs in the whole body through nerves and vessels, and the individuality of people with reference to age, sex, temperament, idiosyncrasy, etc. (7)

Reil then defines his scientific approach to pharmacology:

> The only way pharmacology can improve is to carry out tests, note the results carefully and subsume the isolated observations into higher-level rules... at the same time this will serve to explain the effects of drugs... Now I have stated above that we are not able to explain the action of drugs because we do not know their

composition or the disposition of the human body in sickness or in health, or how they act on one another....Until now an explanation of how drugs work, and therefore a science-based pharmacological discipline has not been possible. The way forward is clear, namely: a) painstaking research into the nature of drugs, especially their composition; b) research into physiology and especially animal chemistry; c) accurate observation of what happens in the interaction between drugs and the human body and an accurate integration of these phenomena into higher rules. All other methods are wrong and all attempts to find a principle to explain these things in any other way is a waste of time. (7)

To complete his scientific approach to pharmacology, Reil presents a set of eight rules for the evaluation of drugs and these merit closer study. (7-9)

Reil's Rules

As his first rule, Reil chooses to emphasise the overall approach and motivation for pharmacological research and indeed for any form of scientific endeavour.

1) The observer must have good common sense, good understanding, judgement, know how to make observations but also have a healthy degree of scepticism. He should not allow himself to be influenced by egotism, doctrine, an attachment to his school, or any prejudice, but by the simple love of truth.

Next, he states the importance of standardization both in respect to the drug under test and to the research participants. He notes that the researcher has the power to control the quality and consistency of drugs used, but the inter and intra-individual variation of human subjects can only be acknowledged and taken into account.

> 2) If the results of experiments, that is the changes brought about in the human body by the drugs, are consistent, they can be considered to be undoubtedly valid only if both the drugs and the human beings used in the series of tests are of a standardized nature.

His third rule focuses on a similar theme, but here he discusses the importance of accurate diagnosis and previews one of his later themes — the all-importance of consistent nomenclature.

> 3) If we are experimenting on invalids the same things apply. Their illness must not be hypothetical, but real, identifiable from recognizable symptoms and deemed by the experimenter as really being present... How many mistakes have wormed their way into pharmacology because of confused terms about the nature of diseases and an imperfect semiotic of the same.

The reproducibility of research findings is emphasized in Reil's fourth rule. The confounding effects of variables that have not been controlled and the cherry-picking of the desired result from a variety of non-standardised experiments are, in Reil's opinion, reasons for the mistaken advocacy of ineffective treatments.

> 4) The experiments must be repeated often and under exactly the same conditions and in each repetition the results have to be the same. This alone can convince us that the results are effects of the drug.

As an extension to his call for the control of variables within an experiment, Reil makes a call for the study of individual, or simple, drugs in his fifth rule. Here, he draws an important distinction between the study of drugs and their practical use, with his realization that compounds or mixtures will be prescribed. He argues, however, for their components to be tested first separately, and only when understood to be tested in combinations.

> 5) A drug must be tested on its own, not in conjunction with others, because otherwise it remains uncertain which of the substances used has brought about the effect in question... First of all, we must determine the powers of the simple, individual substances in order to be able to work out the effect of compounds of them.

The terminology we use to describe drug actions is called into question by Reil in his sixth rule. Here, he calls for specificity and a greater depth to our language that goes beyond mere superficial description.

> 6) The effects of drugs must be described specifically, not in terms that are too general, as otherwise they are of no practical use.

In Reil's seventh rule, he states the importance of the scientific method in the study of pharmacology. The critical importance of experiential learning and the process of inductive logic are emphasized.

> 7) The effects of drugs must be established either through direct experience or from conclusions, which were clearly able to be drawn from direct experience. Their characteristics have to be clearly described... Isolated observations must be collated and general results deduced according to certain rules (e.g. frequency, causality).

In Reil's eighth and final rule, he returns to his call for improved terminology, with greater precision in the words we use to describe our experimental findings. After stating his rule, he goes on to offer a number of specific examples in support of his argument for a dedicated, technical language of pharmacology.

> 8) Finally, the terminology used in pharmacology deserves sharp criticism. The meaning we give to words needs to be more precise, more expansive and more accurate. Without this improvement we will remain virtually unintelligible to each other.

Although Reil is today remembered for his contributions to medicine, especially neurology and psychiatry, his work in pharmacology, albeit its theoretical basis is less widely acknowledged than it should be. However, not surprisingly, Reil was not alone in asking for a more systematic approach to the study of drug action at that time. In 1799, the same year that he had published his rules, his contemporary Adolph Friedrich Nolde also presented his ideas on the subject.

Nolde's Rules

Adolph Friedrich Nolde was the Professor of Medicine at Rostock, and in his 1799 *Erinnerung an einige zur kritischen Würdigung der Arzneymittel sehr nothwendige Bedingungen* [Reminder of some of the necessary conditions for the critical appraisal of a drug], he also defines and enumerates a set of eight rules for the conduct of pharmacological research. (10) In the first seven of these rules, Nolde highlights the need for the study of high quality and 'genuine and unadulterated' drugs that are 'prescribed in an appropriate manner.' He recognizes that patients with well-characterised diseases must be studied and that any evaluation of new and untested drugs should be done 'with the greatest caution.' He emphasizes the need 'to observe precisely the changes, which are induced by the application of a drug, and investigate properly whether they are caused by it or might be due to other precipitating factors' and 'to repeat our experiments frequently under similar and probably occasionally also under dissimilar conditions.' (10)

Although he covers much the same ground as Reil, it is his eighth rule that merits closest examination. Here, uniquely, he looks at the issue of research misconduct and the impact it may have both on scientific endeavour and the well-being of patients.

He summarises this rule as follows:

> Rule 8. When announcing a new drug or recommending a known drug nothing at all should be omitted about anything that could have an influence on the correct assessment of the drug, and it would be shameful if observations were to be fabricated or distorted at the expense of the truth. (10)

Nolde justifies the inclusion of such a rule by noting that, 'unfortunately one sees many a result which has been recorded untruthfully,' and goes on to state that, 'not everything which physicians publish under the promising titles of "Observations and Experiences" can be taken at face value.' (10) What might be seen as very much a 21st century problem appears to have been a well-recognised phenomenon even in the 18th.

Overall, like Reil, Nolde would have preferred the application of defined pharmacological principles in determining a drug's mechanism of action, but conceded that experimentation might be a necessary first step when he states,

> As long as we cannot specify a drug's mechanism of action according to a Principle of Causality, as long as we have no other choice than that ... we may abstract, with the utmost care and circumspection, through observations and experiences the law by which the drug seems to be working.

Physiology meets pharmacology

Rules for appropriate experimentation can only take us so far. Those rules must be put into practice and while there had been many experiments performed to test the safety and efficacy of drugs, the first that might truly be called formal experimental pharmacology was probably performed in Paris in 1809, a decade after Reil and Nolde had published their works.

The physician responsible was François Magendie (1783-1855). (fig. 4.2) Magendie grew up in post revolutionary France and, although gifted, his education was somewhat piecemeal. He graduated in medicine in 1808 and the following year he wrote:

> '[The] majority of physiological facts must be verified by new experiments and this is the only means of bringing the physics of living bodies out of the state of imperfection in which it lies at present.' (11)

This emphasis on meticulous experimentation led him to investigate the mechanism of action of a series of poisons. The poisonous sap of the Javanese Upas Tree, the Indian Nux Vomica, and the closely related St Ignatius Bean had all at some time been used as arrow poisons. In 1809, Magendie and his colleague Alire Raffeneau-Delille (1778-1850), who was a botanist and physician, presented the results of a series of animal experiments designed to define their mechanism of action. (12) All three plants produced similar pharmacological effects — tetanus and convulsions — and through careful neurological studies Magendie and his colleague showed conclusively that the preparations were acting on the spinal cord. Magendie also concluded that such poisons were absorbed into the bloodstream, rather than the lymphatics, before being transported to their site of action.

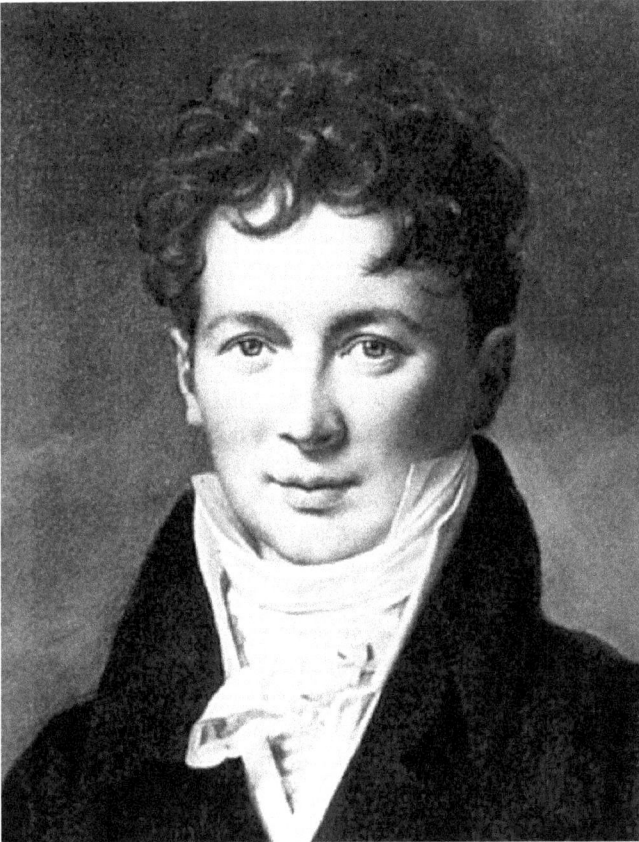

Figure 4.2. François Magendie (1783-1855) c1812. Detail of a painting by Guérin. (Public Domain)

Importantly, Magendie believed that the pharmacological properties of plants were due to their chemical composition and that it should be possible to isolate the active ingredient from a preparation of the plant. This theory was put to the test some years later when, in 1817, Magendie working with the French chemist Pierre-Joseph Pelletier (1788-1842) isolated the active ingredient of the emetic ipecacuanha root, which Pelletier named emetine. (13) The pharmacological properties of this isolate were first confirmed in animal experiments and then human studies. Indeed, in their paper, Magendie and Pelletier wrote,

> One of the memoir's authors did not hesitate at all in taking two grains of emetine himself. Following his example, several young students in medicine also took some, and soon they were all stricken, like the animals, by attacks of vomiting, and by a desire to sleep which disappeared, without leaving any trace of discomfort or indisposition. (14, quoted in translation 15)

The same year Pelletier began a long and highly successful collaboration with another chemist and pharmacist, who had in fact been one of the 'several young students of medicine' in the emetine study: Joseph-Bienaimé Caventou (1795-1877). (15) In 1818, the new team of Pelletier and Caventou isolated strychnine from the St Ignatius Bean in accord with Magendie's prediction. They then went on to isolate a series of alkaloids from plant material including caffeine and colchicine. However, the most important of these isolates was quinine in 1820 from the bark of the Peruvian cinchona tree. (16)

In 1821, Magendie published his own formulary entitled, *Formulaire pour la préparation et l'emploi de plusieurs nouveaux médicaments*. This book was largely based on his own experimental findings and included details of the therapeutic uses of various alkaloids including emetine and strychnine. It was a success, running to nine editions and was translated many times. Indeed, the first use of the word *Formulary* comes from Haden's 1823 English translation of Magendie's *Formulaire*. (17) The publication of the *Formulaire* has even been viewed as marking the beginning of modern pharmacology. (3)

In 1826, Pelletier and Caventou moved into industrial scale production of quinine sulphate when they extracted 1,800 kg from 150 tons of imported cinchona bark. (18) Mass production of medicines of one form or another had occurred before, for example with the preparation of theriac, but this was on a different scale and the purification processes involved meant that this might truly be described as the first step in the creation of a new pharmaceutical industry.

Magendie's pupil Claude Bernard (1813-78) would go on, not only to be his successor in Paris, but also to become one of the greatest of all experimental physiologists. He continued the work that Magendie had begun, working at the interface of physiology and pharmacology and discovered amongst many other things that the arrow poison curare acts at the neuromuscular junction to interrupt the stimulation of muscle by nerve impulses.

Although many view the work of Magendie and Bernard as the beginnings of pharmacology, others argue that they used drugs as little more than reagents in their detailed *in vivo* physiological experiments. For the true beginnings of pharmacology we may have to look elsewhere.

Towards an academic discipline

In 1847, pharmacology took a significant step closer to being a science when Rudolf Buchheim (1820-79) was appointed to the first chair of pharmacology at the University of Dorpat (present day Tartu) in Estonia. (2, 19) (fig. 4.3)

Buchheim, working initially in a pharmacology laboratory he built in the basement of his own home, turned the largely descriptive study of drugs into a modern experimental science. He trained many young physicians and finally established a spacious well-appointed Institute of Pharmacology at the university. Early in his twenty-year tenure at Dorpat he wrote:

> Fortunately, a surgeon who uses the wrong side of the scalpel cuts his own fingers and not the patient; if the same applied to drugs, they would have been investigated very carefully a long time ago. (20)

But, nearer the end of his life, disillusioned with the academic status of pharmacology at the time, Buchheim wrote in 1876,

> Which goal can be reached by a man having devoted himself with all his abilities and efforts to pharmacological research? A professorship with a minimum salary and an empty auditorium! (21)

Buchheim is not credited so much with any fundamental discovery as with the creation of the scientific framework in which pharmacology would develop as a science. This framework consisted of two closely related elements: first that the concept underpinning the classification of drugs should be a 'natural system', based on their mode of action, and second that an experimental approach was needed to unravel these mechanisms of action. Today this approach might seem obvious, but at the time it was radical and highly controversial.

But, perhaps Buchheim's greatest contribution was as a teacher and mentor for it was the achievement of his students that will be his greatest legacy. One student in particular would not only carry his torch but would bring global recognition to the new discipline of pharmacology.

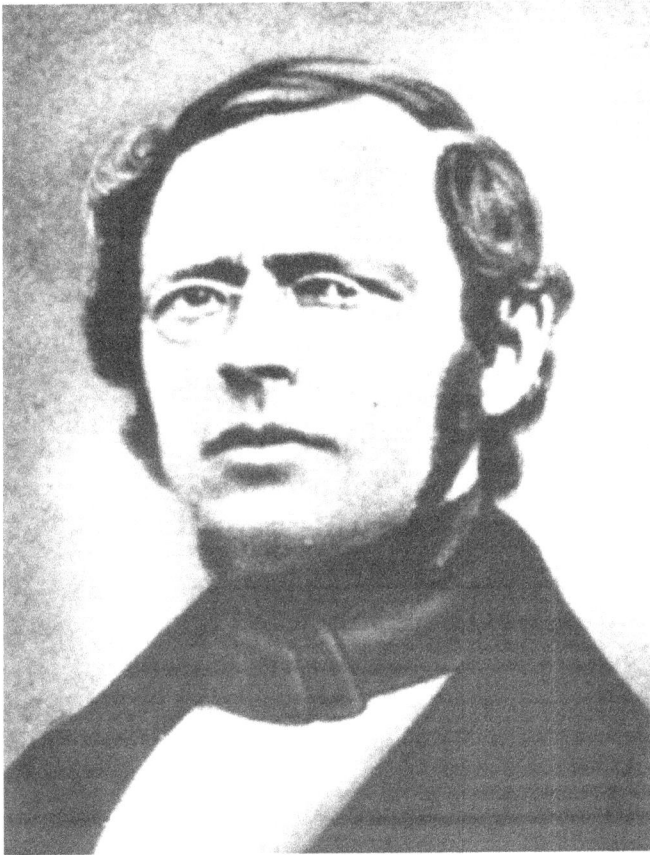

Figure 4.3. Rudolf Buchheim (1820-79), photograph c1850. (Public Domain)

That student was Oswald Schmiedeberg (1838-1921) who completed his thesis on the measurement of chloroform in blood under Buchheim in 1866 and three years later he took over from his supervisor as Professor of Pharmacology. (2) (fig. 4.4) He supplemented his training with a sabbatical year in Leipzig, where he acquired further experimental skills and subsequently moved to the University of Strassbourg in 1872 where he would remain for the rest of his professional life and establish what at the time would be the most important centre for the study of pharmacology in the world.

During a long and highly productive career he made many discoveries and contributed significantly to his developing field. However, like Buchheim, Schmiedeberg was also a mentor and one of his legacies was the training of a whole new generation of pharmacologists who would go on to sit in more than forty chairs in universities around the world. These trainees included John Jacob Abel who would become the first Professor of Pharmacology in the US and the Scotsman Arthur Cushny, who would become Abel's successor and who would have such an important role to play in developing Departments of Pharmacology in the UK. (22) Today, it is Schmiedeberg rather than Buchheim who is regarded as the father of modern pharmacology, but Schmiedeberg himself was always the first to acknowledge the debt he owed his former professor.

The debt, however, that both men and the developing science of pharmacology owed to Reil, Nolde and others like them remains largely unacknowledged. Nevertheless, without physicians of the enlightenment such as these, who questioned the status quo and called for the application of scientific rigour, it is hard to imagine that pharmacology as we understand it today could have developed, and flourished to become one of the central pillars of modern medicine.

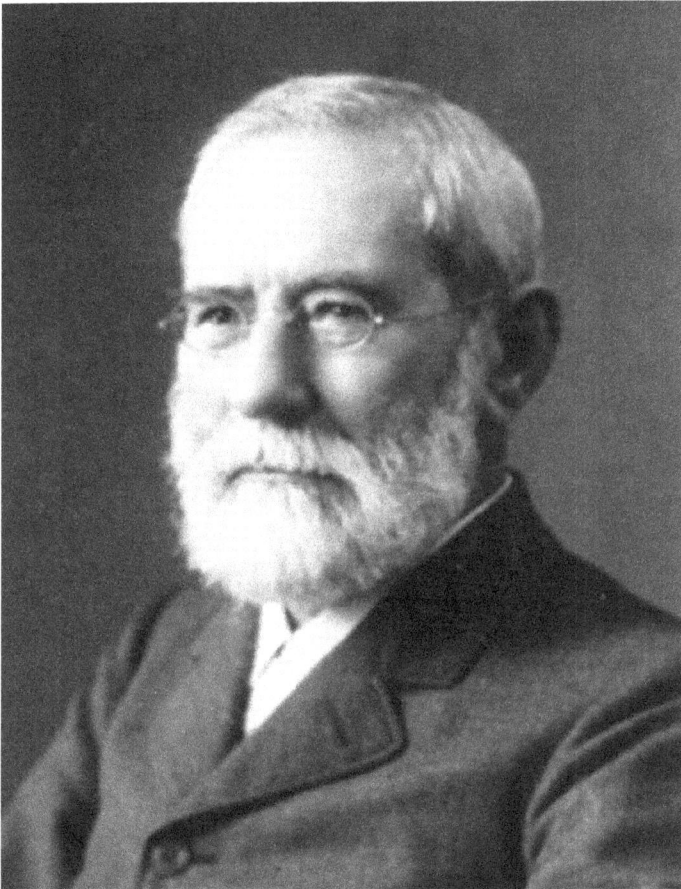

Figure 4.4. Oswald Schmiedeberg (1838–1921), photograph c1900. (Public Domain)

Conclusions

In Europe, during the late 18th and early 19th centuries, we can chart a series of beginnings. We have eminent German Professors of Medicine picking up where Galen and Avicenna had left off and proposing new investigative frameworks for the study of drugs; we have pharmacology emerging from the interdisciplinary overlap between medicine, physiology and chemistry and developing as an academic discipline in its own right; and we have the development of organic chemistry. The latter allowed the extraction and isolation of the active pharmacological ingredients of well-known herbal remedies and poisons for the first time. Physiologists could now turn their attentions to the effects of these isolates and begin to define mechanisms of action and to suggest therapeutic uses. In so doing, they became pharmacologists.

Thus far, however, these scientists have only been able to refine what nature has already provided. The next step will be to synthesise new molecules and to study their pharmacology and clinical application. The era of drug discovery is almost upon us.

References

1. Bonner TN. *Becoming a Physician: Medical Education in Great Britain, France, Germany, and the United States, 1750-1945.* Oxford University Press, Oxford, 1995.

2. Muscholl E. The evolution of experimental pharmacology as a biological science: the pioneering work of Buchheim and Schmiedeberg. *British Journal of Pharmacology* 1995; 116: 2155-9.

3. Bickel MH. [The development of experimental pharmacology 1790-1850]. *Gesnerus Supplement* 2000; 46: 7-158.

4. Anon. Johann Christian Reil (1759-1813) *The Dictionary of*

Eighteenth Century German Philosophers. Eds Kuehn M, Klemme H, Continuum, London, 2010.

5. Binder DK, Schaller K, Clusmann H. The seminal contributions of Johann-Christian Reil to anatomy, physiology, and psychiatry. *Neurosurgery* 2007; 61: 1091-6.

6. Marneros A. Psychiatry's 200th birthday. *British Journal of Psychiatry* 2008; 193: 1-3.

7. Reil JC. Beitrag zu den Prinzipien für jede künftige Pharmakologie. *Röschlands Magazin* 1799; 3: 26-64.

8. Kästner I. Reil's "Beitrag zu den Prinzipien für jede künftige Pharmakologie" In: *Johann Christian Reil (1759-1813): Hallesches Symposium 1988* Eds Kaiser W, Völker A. Halle (Saale): Martin-Luther-Universität Halle-Wittenberg 1989.

9. Gaw A. 'The principles of a future pharmacology': Johann Christian Reil (1759-1813) and his role in the development of clinical pharmacology. *European Journal of Clinical Pharmacology* 2016; 72: 13-7.

10. Nolde AF. Erinnerung an einige zur kritischen Würdigung der Arzneymittel sehr nothwendige Bedingungen. [Reminder of some of the necessary conditions for the critical appraisal of a drug.] *Hufelands Journal* 1799; 8: 1. St. S. 47-97, 2. St. S. 75-116.

11. Magendie F. Quelques idées générales sur les phénomènes particuliers aux corps vivans. *Bulletin des Sciences Médicales de la Societé Médicale d'Emulation de Paris* 1809; 4: 145-70.

12. Magendie F, Raffeneau-Delille A. Examen de l'action de quelques végétaux sur la moelle épinière. *Nouveau Bulletin Scientifique de la Société Philomatique* 1809; 1: 368-405.

13. Pelletier PJ, Magendie F. Recherches chimiques et physiologiques sur l'ipecacuanha. *Annales de Chimie et de Physique* 1817; 4: 172-85.

14. Magendie F, Pelletier, PJ. Sur l'Emétine, et sur les trois espèces d'Ipécacuanha. *Journal général de médecine de chirurgie et de pharmacie Françaises et étrangères ou recueil périodique de la Société de Médecine de Paris* 1817; 59: 223-31.

15. Simon J. Naming and toxicity: a history of Strychnine *Studies in History and Philosophy of Biological and Biomedical Sciences* 1999; 30: 505-25.

16. Pelletier PJ, Caventou JB. Recherches chimiques sur les quinquinas. *Annales de Chimie et de Physique* 1820; 15: 289-318 & 337-65.

17. Aronson J. Formularies and pharmacopoeias. *British Medical Journal* 2011; 342: d34.

18. Raviña E. *The Evolution of Drug Discovery: From Traditional Medicines to Modern Drugs.* Wiley-VCH, Weinheim, 2011.

19. Habermann ER. Rudolf Buchheim and the beginning of pharmacology as a science. *Annual Review of Pharmacology* 1974; 14: 1-9.

20. Buchheim R. *Beitrage zur Arzneimittellehre.* Voss, Leipzig, 1849.

21. Buchheim R. Ueber die Aufgaben und die Stellung der Pharmakologie an den deutschen Hochschulen. *Archiv for Experimentelle Pathologie und Pharmakologie* 1876; 5: 261-78.

22. Parascandola J. Reflections on the history of pharmacology. *Trends in Pharmacological Sciences* 1982; March: 93-4.

——— ∎ ———

5

Two Weeks that Shook
the Medical World

The Beginnings of Drug
Synthesis

Introduction

For most of our story so far, drugs have been derived from
plants and minerals. While active compounds may have been
extracted from crude preparations, there had been little
attempt to manipulate the naturally occurring molecules with a
view to enhancing or altering their pharmacological function.
This was soon to change and as our expertise in organic
chemistry advanced so did our realization that the route to new
drugs may be through the manipulation of existing ones. In

this chapter, we will look at how two of the most famous drugs in history were synthesized from older already well-established treatments at the same laboratory bench by the same man within a fortnight.

Salicylic acid

This story begins with Herr Hoffmann's rheumatism. During the 1890s this German industrialist had been suffering badly and had been medicating himself with salicylic acid — the standard treatment of the day. However, while this drug soothed his pains, it had significant side effects, including gastric irritation, nausea and tinnitus. Moreover, it had a terribly bitter taste making it almost unpalatable for daily use. (1)

He complained to his son Felix and asked him if an alternative could be found. His son was Dr Felix Hoffmann, who at the time was a 29-year old chemist working for the German pharmaceutical company, Friedrich Bayer & Co in Elberfeld, now part of Wuppertal, in North Rhine-Westphalia. (2) (fig. 5.1)

Salicylic acid is the active component of the extracts of willow leaves and bark, which have been recommended for the treatment of rheumatism for over 5,000 years. Ancient Egyptian, Greek and Roman medicine were well acquainted with the properties of willow bark extract and there is a long folk-tradition of its use as a treatment for fever and pain. (3) However, it was not until the 18th century that the first clinical trial was conducted, by an amateur English scientist, the Rev. Edward Stone.

Stone was a country parson from Chipping Norton, Oxfordshire who himself suffered from ague or a malarial like fever and shivering. (3, 4) He was aware of the folk use of willow bark for the treatment for such symptoms and while walking one day chanced upon a willow tree and decided to chew a piece of its bark for relief. He noted his surprise 'at its extraordinary bitterness; which immediately raised me a suspicion of its having the properties of the Peruvian bark.' (4) The latter was cinchona bark, from which the drug quinine is extracted. The taste, and the situation of the tree, sparked his interest. He reasoned,

> As this tree delights in a moist or wet soil, where agues chiefly abound, the general maxim, that many natural maladies carry their cures along with them, or that their remedies lie not far from their causes, was so very apposite to this particular case, that I could not help applying it; and that this might be the intention of Providence here, I must own, had some little weight with me. (4)

But, folklore was not enough and he, 'determined to make some experiments with it...' He gathered approximately 500g of the bark, dried and pulverized it and dispersed it in tea, small beer or water and stated, 'It was not long before I had an opportunity of making a trial of it...' (4)

Over a five-year period he administered his extracts to 50 patients with various forms of fever, and experimented with the most effective dose, concluding that 1 dram (1.8g) cured their fever.
He submitted his findings to the Royal Society for publication in April 1763 concluding,

> I have no other motives for publishing this valuable specific, than that it may have a fair and full trial in all its variety of circumstances and situations, and that the world may reap the benefits accruing from it. (4)

Almost a century later his hopes were realized when the active component of willow bark, salicylic acid, was first chemically synthesized in 1860 by the German chemist, Hermann Kolbe.

(5) This breakthrough made the large-scale industrial synthesis of the drug possible by 1874 and led to its widespread use, including that of Felix Hoffmann's father.

Aspirin

In 1897, Felix Hoffmann was working in a newly established chemistry and pharmacology laboratory at Bayer under the leadership of Heinrich Dreser. (fig. 5.2)

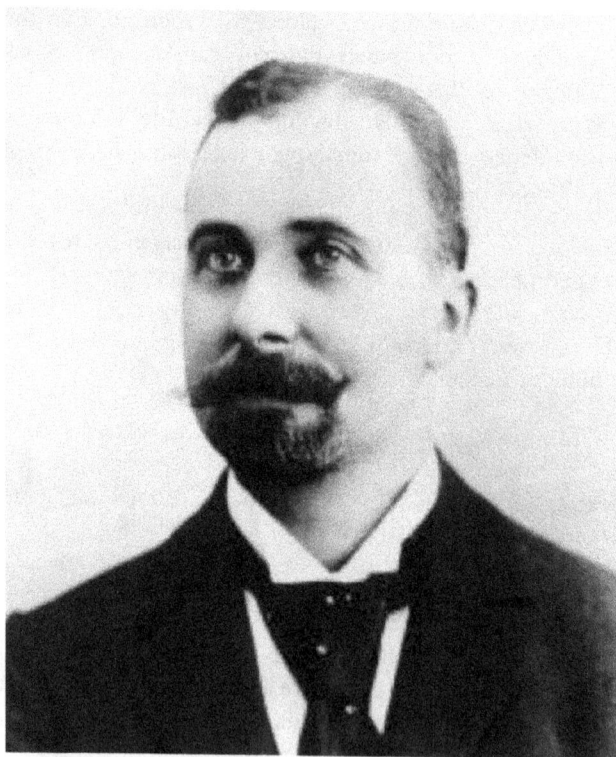

Figure 5.1 Felix Hoffmann (1868-1946), photograph c1900. (Courtesy of Bayer: Public Domain)

Dreser was a highly methodical researcher who is credited with introducing large-scale animal testing to the pharmaceutical industry. But he was also an astute businessman who could see the commercial potential of exciting new products.

On Tuesday, 10 August 1897 Hoffmann, at his laboratory bench in Elberfeld, modified salicylic acid and synthesized the derivative acetylsalicylic acid. (fig. 5.3) This was subsequently tested in animal studies and found to have anti-inflammatory, analgesic and antipyretic properties. After initially dismissing it because of concerns that it may have cardiac side-effects, Dreser was eventually persuaded of the huge commercial opportunity that acetylsalicylic acid offered and it was brought to market in 1899 under the trade name Aspirin, first as a powder and then as tablets. (2, 6) The drug quickly found favour and it has been in continuous use for more than century.

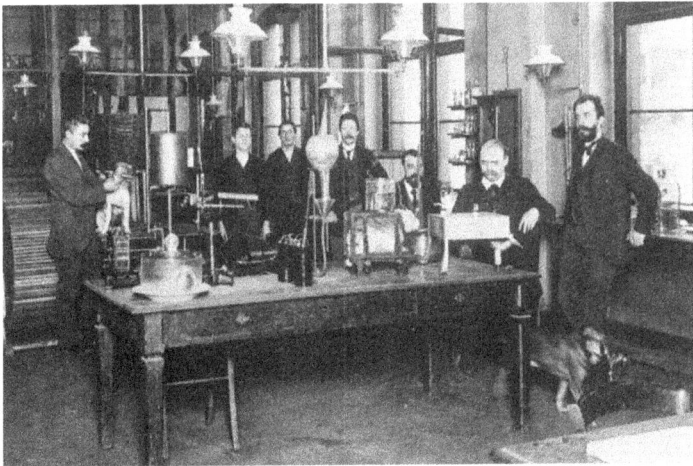

Figure 5.2 Heinrich Dreser (1860-1924) (seated second from right) in the Bayer Pharmacology Laboratory, photograph 1897. (Courtesy of Bayer: Public Domain)

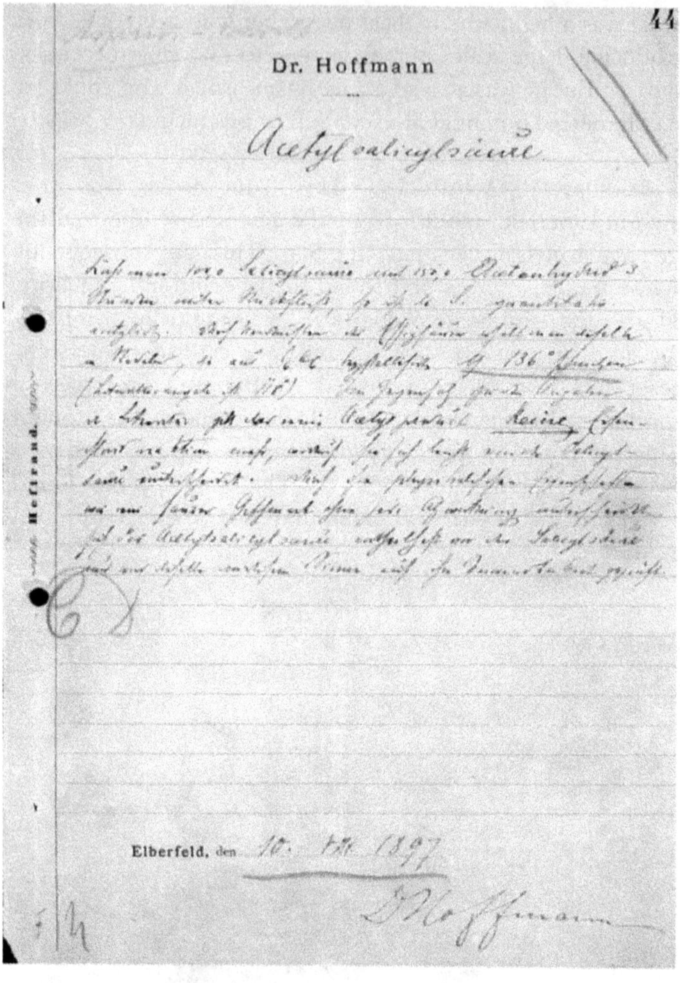

Dr. Hoffmann

Acetylsalicylsäure

Elberfeld, den 10. VIII. 1897

Figure 5.3 Page from Felix Hoffmann's laboratory book from 10 August 1897, the day he first synthesized acetylsalicylic acid. (Courtesy of Bayer: Public Domain)

Acetylsalicylic acid received its trade name, Aspirin, from Dreser (7), but there are two schools of thought about why he chose this name (1). Meadowsweet is a plant that contains salicylaldehyde, which can be oxidized to salicylic acid. The genus name of this herb is *Spirea* and thus the German name for the acid derived from it was Spirsäure and its acetylated form, Acetylspirsäure, which could easily be truncated to Aspirin. Rather more romantically, he may have known about the patron saint of headaches St Aspirinius and named his new analgesic after him.

This account of Aspirin's invention has, however, recently been challenged as a piece of Nazi revisionist history. (8) Perhaps the true inventor of Aspirin was the Jewish chemist Arthur Eichengrün (1867-1949) (fig. 5.4), who claimed while he was interred in Theresienstadt concentration camp and afterwards that Hoffmann had been working under him at the time and that he had led the clinical experiments (many of which were surreptitious) to examine the effectiveness of acetylsalicylic acid that had led to it being brought to market in 1899. (9)

Bayer have refuted this claim, pointing out that Eichengrün was not Hoffmann's superior (they were almost exact contemporaries) and citing the US Patent for Aspirin which was clearly submitted in 1900 in the name of Felix Hoffmann. (fig. 5.5) The relevant text reads,

> Be it known that I, FELIX HOFFMANN, doctor of philosophy, chemist, (assignor to the FARBENFABRIKEN on ELBERFELD COMPANY, of New York,) residing at Elberfeld, Germany, have invented a new and useful Improvement in the Manufacture or Production of Acetyl Salicylic Acid; and I hereby declare the following to be a clear and exact description of my invention.

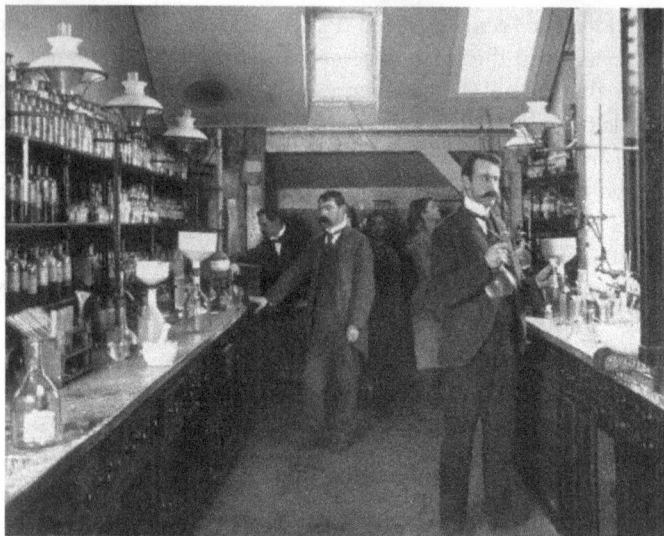

Figure 5.4 Arthur Eichengrün (1867-1949) (in foreground) in the Bayer Pharmacology Laboratory c1900. (Courtesy of Bayer: Public Domain)

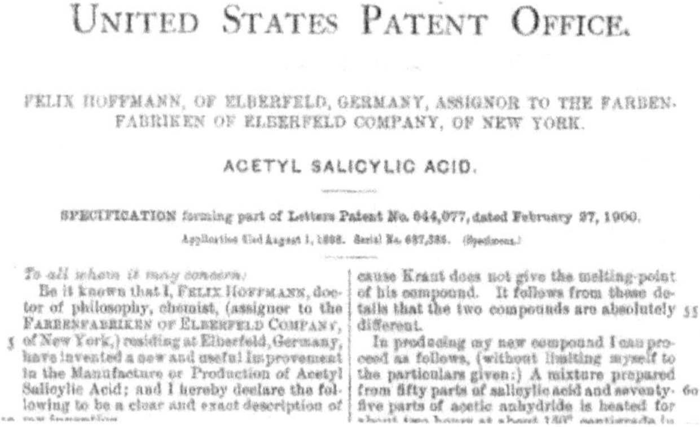

UNITED STATES PATENT OFFICE.

FELIX HOFFMANN, OF ELBERFELD, GERMANY, ASSIGNOR TO THE FARBEN-FABRIKEN OF ELBERFELD COMPANY, OF NEW YORK.

ACETYL SALICYLIC ACID.

SPECIFICATION forming part of Letters Patent No. 644,077, dated February 27, 1900.

Application filed August 1, 1898. Serial No. 687,385. (Specimens.)

To all whom it may concern:

Be it known that I, FELIX HOFFMANN, doctor of philosophy, chemist, (assignor to the FARBENFABRIKEN OF ELBERFELD COMPANY,) of New York,) residing at Elberfeld, Germany, have invented a new and useful Improvement in the Manufacture or Production of Acetyl Salicylic Acid; and I hereby declare the following to be a clear and exact description of my invention:

cause Kraut does not give the melting-point of his compound. It follows from these details that the two compounds are absolutely different.

In producing my new compound I can proceed as follows, (without limiting myself to the particulars given:) A mixture prepared from fifty parts of salicylic acid and seventy-five parts of acetic anhydride is heated for about two hours at about 150° centigrade in

Figure 5.5 US Patent application designating Felix Hoffmann as the inventor of acetylsalicylic acid, dated 27 February 1900. (Public Domain)

94

At the time of the submission, Eichengrün was still a Bayer employee and if his later story were true why was the issue not raised then?

Whatever the truth of the matter, Bayer's fortunes were to be built on the launch of one of the most widely used drugs in history. In 2000, it was estimated that fifty thousand tons of acetylsalicylic acid are produced annually and that the average consumption is 80 tablets per person per year. (3)

However, it would be another 70 years before we would understand how Aspirin worked. In 1971, the British pharmacologist John Vane discovered the mechanism by which aceyltsalicylic acid exerts its anti-inflammatory, analgesic and antipyretic actions. (3) He showed that Aspirin, and other non-steroidal anti-inflammatory drugs (NSAIDs), inhibit the activity of cyclo-oxygenase (COX), the enzyme which leads to the formation of prostaglandins that cause inflammation, swelling, pain and fever. (1) For this work he was jointly awarded the 1982 Nobel Prize in Physiology or Medicine.

But, Hoffmann's work that summer of 1897 was not over yet.

Opiates

The process of acetylation had been used before and would be again in order to alter a natural compound's structure in the hope of either enhancing its efficacy or minimizing its side effects. Perhaps because of Hoffmann's success with salicylic acid, Dreser asked him to work on another compound just a few days later. Dreser was known to keep a keen eye on the literature and regularly searched through archives in the hope of turning up a new and commercially viable line of research. Twenty-three years earlier the English chemist CR Alder Wright, working at St Mary's in London had been experimenting with morphine. (10) He had acetylated it and, although he did not pursue the development of the product, he did publish his preliminary findings, which Dreser had uncovered. Opium had of course been in use for millennia and its most abundant active component, morphine, had been extracted in around 1804 by a young apprentice pharmacist, Friedrich Wilhelm Sertürner (1783-1841). (11)

While working as an assistant in a Pharmacy in Paderborn, Germany, Sertürner was the first to isolate an active principle from any plant material when he isolated what was to become known as morphine from the juice of the opium poppy. There is debate over the exact date of his isolation, but Sertürner initially published his work in 1806 (12), not in an academic journal but in what was effectively a trade magazine for German apothecaries. (13, 14) As such, his discovery remained unrecognized by the scientific community for a decade. Sertürner published further details of his work in other articles and eventually in a more prominent journal. (15) It was the French chemist and physicist Joseph Louis Gay-Lussac (1778-1850) who rediscovered Sertürner's work, translated his paper into French and published it along with an editorial in the prestigious *Annales de Chimie* in 1817. (16)

In his 1817 paper, Sertürner described his chemical isolation techniques and his experiments on animals as well as those on human subjects, including himself. He self-administered increasing doses of his isolate and enlisted the help of three 17-year-old friends. He noted,

> A general redness, which could even be seen in the eyes, covered their faces, principally the cheeks, and the vital forces seemed exalted. (15)

All four were effectively suffering from morphine poisoning as they had ingested large doses. Because he had experienced a dream-like sleep while dosed with his opium extract, Sertürner decided to name it *morphium* after Morpheus the Greek god of dreams. When Gay-Lussac translated Sertürner's paper he changed this to *morphine* in an attempt to standardize the nomenclature of organic plant alkalis, or alkaloids as they would become known the following year. (14)

Heroin

After morphine, the second most abundant active component in opium, 3-methylmorphine or *codeine*, was isolated in 1832 by the French chemist and pharmacologist Pierre Jean Robiquet. (17)   Dreser had previously worked on the chemistry of codeine and, like all in the pharmaceutical industry at the time, he was keen to develop new non-addictive alternatives to these opiates. Perhaps, acetylation would do the trick.

On Saturday 21 August 1897, at the same bench where just over ten days before he had successfully acetylated salicylic acid to produce Aspirin, Felix Hoffmann was working on morphine. He used Wright's method to add two acetyl groups and produced diacetyl morphine or as it has become known diamorphine — the drug that Bayer would subsequently market under the trade name Heroin. The name derived from the German word *heroisch*, meaning heroic or great — which was how those Bayer employees who sampled the new drug reported their feelings. (18) The demand for a safer opiate at the time had little to do with pain relief, but more to do with cough suppression.   This was the age of tuberculosis and various other respiratory problems and debilitating coughs were a significant clinical problem.

The Bayer chemists found that Heroin was more potent than morphine or codeine, but concluded erroneously that it was associated with less respiratory depression. (14) In 1898, it was brought to market as a safer, more potent cough suppressant and advertising of the time emphasized this indication. Within 12 months of its launch, Bayer was manufacturing a ton of Heroin a year and exporting it to more than 20 countries. (19) (fig. 5.6)

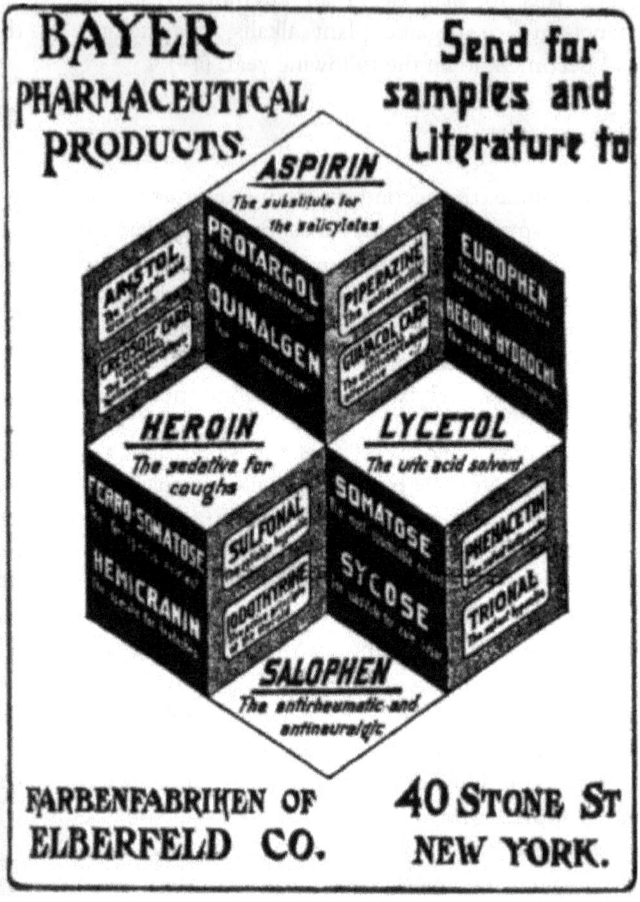

Figure 5.6 Bayer composite US advertisement for several of its products, including Aspirin and Heroin c1900. (Public Domain)

Almost immediately the drug created controversy with one clinician claiming it to be 'the digitalis of the respiration' and another an 'extremely dangerous poison.' (8)   Time would reveal the highly addictive properties of Heroin and result in its restricted use or complete ban.

The success of these drugs and the story behind their invention prompts an important question.   Who actually invented Aspirin and Heroin?

Both drugs had been synthesized before 1897.   Acetylsalicylic acid had been produced in France in 1853 by the French chemist Charles Frédéric Gerhardt (20) and later by German chemists who correctly worked out its chemical structure, while diacetyl morphine had first been synthesized in England in 1874 by the English chemist CR Alder Wright. (10)

However, at least in the case of acetylsalicylic acid, the method used by Hoffmann resulted in a purer, more stable form of the drug.   Moreover, it was the realization in the Bayer laboratory of their commercial potential that transformed two relatively insubstantial reports of organic synthesis into blockbuster products.

While Hoffmann is credited with their synthesis at the laboratory bench during that remarkable summer of 1897 and while Eichengrün was undoubtedly involved to some extent, it is hard to imagine that either drug would have reached the market in quite the way they did without the influence of Dreser, who may be seen as the driving force behind both drugs.   Thus, it is Heinrich Dreser who can perhaps rightly claim to be the true inventor of both Aspirin and Heroin.

Aftermath

What became of Dreser, Hoffmann and Eichengrün? Dreser's contract with Bayer allowed him to benefit financially from the sales of the drugs that he developed and as such he became very wealthy and retired early. Some claim that he became addicted to one of his own drugs — Heroin — and he died aged 64 in Switzerland. (19)

Hoffmann was promoted, and shortly after his productive summer of 1897 he was made head of the pharmaceutical marketing department, where he remained until his retirement. To move one of your most creative organic chemists from the lab where he had synthesized not one but two of the most important drugs in history, to a desk in a marketing department seems a strange decision — at least to anyone who has not worked in the modern pharmaceutical industry where such restructurings and redeployments are bewilderingly commonplace. Hoffmann too died in Switzerland, aged 78. (21)

Eichengrün left Bayer in 1908 to set up his own highly successful pharmaceutical and chemical company and he held over 40 patents. A Jewish industrialist working in Nazi Germany, he naturally came into conflict with the authorities and spent some time in a concentration camp where he made his initial claims of his involvement with the development of Aspirin. He pursued this on his release and published a detailed account shortly before his death in 1949 at the age of 82. (9)

Interestingly, while there has been a lengthy dispute over claims to the invention of Aspirin, there has never been the same scramble to take credit for Heroin. What is not in doubt is that both drugs began their commercial futures on a laboratory bench in Elberfeld during two summer weeks in 1897. Their impacts on human suffering, both as a relief and as a cause have since been incalculable.

Conclusions

With the addition of a functional side group, Hoffmann was able to transform two well-known and well-established, although imperfect, treatments into new drugs. His efforts and those of the many other chemists working at similar laboratory benches across the world led to an explosion of new compounds, a small number of which would ultimately make it to the pharmacy shelves.

As we move from the simple extraction of pharmacologically active compounds from plants and other natural sources to the manipulation of those molecules to create new drugs we enter a new phase of discovery. And it is that era of drug discovery that we will explore in the next chapter.

References

1.   Vane JR, Botting RM. The mechanism of action of aspirin. *Thrombosis Research* 2003; 110: 255-8.

2.   Sneader W. The discovery of aspirin: a reappraisal. *British Medical Journal* 2000; 321: 1591-4.

3.   Vane JR. The fight against rheumatism: from willow bark to COX-1 sparing drugs. *Journal of Physiology and Pharmacology* 2000; 51: 573-86.

4.   Stone E. An account of the success of the bark of the willow in the cure of the agues. *Philosophical Transactions of the Royal Society* 1763; 53: 195-200.

5.   Kolbe H. Ueber Synthese der Salicylsäure. *Annalen der Chemie und Pharmacie* 1860; 113: 125-27.

6.   Chemical Heritage Foundation
      http://www.chemheritage.org/discover/online-

resources/chemistry-in-
history/themes/pharmaceuticals/relieving-
symptoms/hoffmann.aspx (Accessed 8 January 2016)

7.   Dreser H. Pharmacologisches über Aspirin (Acetylsalicyl-
        säure). *Pflügers Archiv* 1899; 76: 306-18.

8.   de Ridder M. Heroin: new facts about an old myth. *Journal of
        Psychoactive Drugs* 1994; 26: 65-8.

9.   Eichengrün A. 50 Jahre Aspirin. *Pharmazie* 1949; 4: 582-4.

10.   Wright CRA. On the action of organic acids and their
        anhydrides on the natural alkaloids: part I. *Journal of the
        Chemical Society* 1874; 27: 1031-42.

11.   Schmitz R. Friedrich Wilhelm Sertürner and the discovery of
        morphine. *Pharmacy in History* 1985; 27: 61-74.

12.   Sertürner FW. Darstellung der reinen Mohnsäure
        (Opiumsäure) nebst einer Chemischen Untersuchung des
        Opiums mit vorzüglicher Hinsicht auf einen darin neu
        entdeckten Stoff und die dahin gehörigen Bemerkungen. *J
        Pharmacie für Aerzte und Apotheker* 1806; 14: 47-93.

13.   Raviña E. *The Evolution of Drug Discovery: From Traditional
        Medicines to Modern Drugs.* Wiley-VCH, Weinheim, 2011.

14.   Sneader W. The discovery of heroin. *Lancet* 1998; 352: 1697-9.

15.   Sertürner FW. Ueber das Morphium, eine neue salzfähige
        Grundlage, und die Mekonsäure, als Hauptbestandtheile des
        Opium. *Annalen der Physik* 1817; 55: 56-89.

16.   Sertürner FW. Analyse de l'Opium. De la Morphine et de
        l'Acide méconique, considérés comme parties essentielles de
        l'opium. *Annales de chimie et de physique* 1817; 5: 26-7.

17.   Miller RJ, Tran PB. More mysteries of opium reveal'd: 300
        years of opiates. *Trends in Pharmacological Sciences* 2000; 21: 299-
        304.

18.   Scott I. Heroin: A hundred-year habit. *History Today* 1998; 46. http://www.historytoday.com/ian-scott/heroin-hundred-year-habit (Accessed 8 January 2016)

19.   Askwith R. How aspirin turned hero. *Sunday Times* 13 September 1998.

20.   Gerhardt C. Untersuchungen über die wasserfreien organischen Säuren. *Annalen der Chemie und Pharmacie* 1853; 87: 149-79.

21.   Bayer. Biographies: Felix Hoffmann. http://www.bayer.com/en/felix-hoffmann.aspx (Accessed 8 January 2016)

——— ■ ———

6

Magic Bullets

The Beginnings of Drug
Discovery

Introduction

Superstition claims that you can charm a bullet so that it will hit only your intended target and nothing else. Such specificity of attack would clearly be of advantage in the confusion of battle, but it also has an attraction when we think about drug treatments. Many, if not most, drugs are poisons. If we could ensure that their actions were targeted, leading to a defined and limited therapeutic response without collateral damage, we would be a long way towards achieving our therapeutic goals.

This notion of a 'magic bullet' was coined by the German clinician and bacteriologist Paul Ehrlich. He first used the term at a lecture in London in 1908 (1), although his concept of *Zauberkugel* had appeared earlier in his writings in German. (2)

Drug discovery in the 20th century has largely been about the search for magic bullets, but this discovery of new drugs takes many forms. While we would like to believe that this is always a process driven by rational and careful scientific method, in reality this is only part of the story. In truth, chance plays as much of a role as innovation.

In this chapter, I want to look at these different threads of discovery, beginning with examples of serendipity, where mistakes have allowed researchers to stumble upon important, new drug treatments. I will also look at how unexpected findings can foster new discoveries, and finally I will look at a more ordered and reasoned approach to drug discovery with the development of receptor theory, the matching of new candidate compounds to validated targets and culminating in the engineering of completely new molecules.

Serendipity

Mistakes, or at least the happy accidents of serendipity, inform and shape drug discovery, just as they have a hand in the development of most human endeavours. There are many examples where the consequences of our errors have led to medical breakthroughs and by examining them we can learn an important lesson about the nature of discovery. Here are just three very different examples.

A new treatment for gunshot wounds

Ambroise Paré was a French barber-surgeon of the 16th century who spent much of his career in military medicine (fig. 6.1). Gunshot wounds, a relatively recent problem on the 16th century battlefield, were believed to be poisonous and they had to be treated, purged and sealed. (3)

Consequently, in war, it was standard practice in Paré's day to cauterise a soldier's wounds with boiling oil. This treatment had been advocated by the established authority in the field, Giovanni da Vigo, the surgeon to the Pope, no less.

In around 1537, while serving under Francis I at the Siege of Turin, Paré used this technique until he ran out of the necessary oil. In an attempt to cleanse and seal the soldiers' wounds, he mixed a cocktail of egg yolk, oil of roses and turpentine and applied this instead. Paré recounts what happened next in his own words.

> That night I could not sleep easily thinking that by the default in cautery I would find the wounded to whom I had failed to apply the said oil dead of poisoning; and this made me get up at first light to visit them. Beyond my hopes I found those on whom I had put the digestive dressing feeling little pain from their wounds which were not swollen or inflamed, and having spent quite a restful night. But the others, to whom the said oil had been applied, I found fevered, with great pain and swelling around their wounds. From then I resolved never again so cruelly to burn poor men wounded with arquebus [a forerunner of the rifle] shot. (Pare 1545, translated in 3)

Forced to reach for an alternative concoction because the standard one was simply unavailable meant Paré had discovered by chance a much better treatment and opened a new chapter in wound care. He went on to publish this highly unorthodox treatment for gunshot wounds in his 'Method of Treating Wounds' in 1545 (4) and revolutionised medical practice in the 16th century.

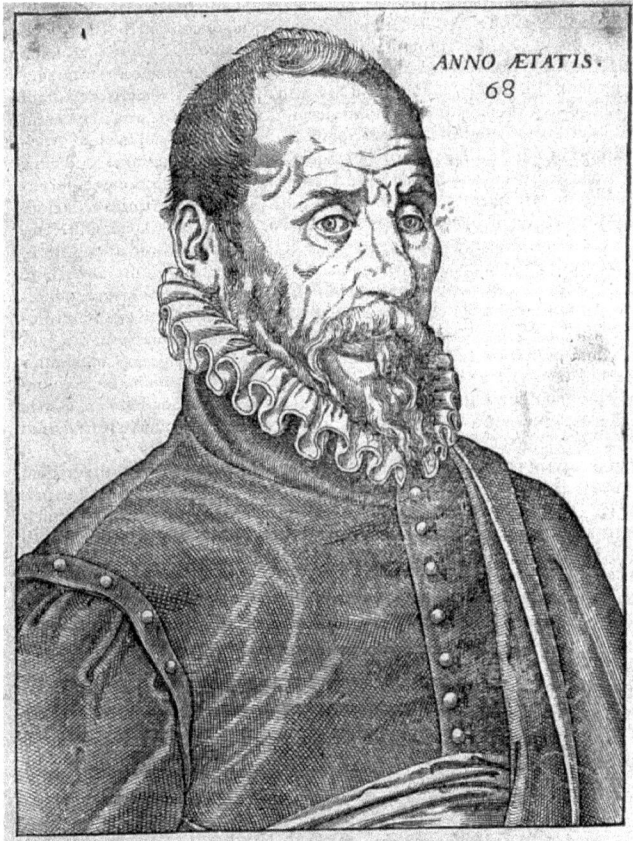

Figure 6.1 Portrait of Ambroise Paré (1510 – 1590). A 1578 woodcut taken from *Opera Ambrosei Pare*, published by Du Puys, Paris, 1582. (Wellcome Library, London)

Such obvious serendipity is not uncommon, especially in an era before any rational approach to therapeutics was possible. Indeed, how else could new drug discovery take place, other than by means of a happy, favourable accident? Certainly not by means of any deliberate drug-hunting strategy or designer-synthesis of new compounds. Apart from the collections of drugs, whose actions had been noted in pre-history and which had been documented over the last three millennia, any new drug would have to be stumbled upon quite by chance.

But, we do not have to confine our examples of serendipity in therapeutics to the distant past. Serendipity has worked just as effectively in the 20th as it has in previous centuries.

The first cancer chemotherapy

Almost 400 years later, the events on another European battlefield would lead to the development of the first anti-cancer drugs. Chemical warfare seems an unlikely place to begin any discussion of drug discovery, but we should never forget the words of Paracelsus, which we encountered in Chapter 1: 'Poison is in everything, and no thing is without poison. The dosage makes it either a poison or a remedy.'

Chemical warfare used in World War I claimed the lives of approximately 90,000 soldiers and accounted for more than 1.3 million casualties. (5) As well as chlorine and phosgene, nitrogen mustard gas was used to attack soldiers in the trenches.

The first report of the haematological side effects of mustard gas came in 1919 from a physician who had been treating exposed soldiers on the Western Front (6). He noted a marked reduction in the circulating white blood cells in these victims. Later, research at Yale School of Medicine, under the leadership of the pharmacologist Alfred Gilman and the physician Louis Goodman, confirmed those early findings and extended the study to the effects of the poison in animal models of lymphoma. (7)

The first human trial was in a single patient suffering from refractory lymphosarcoma. This patient received his first intravenous dose of mustine, a liquid derivative of mustard gas, on 27 August 1942. Despite early regression of his tumours, he suffered the consequences of aplastic anaemia and died on day 96 of his treatment.

Almost exactly one year later, a significant body of data on human exposure to mustard gas was obtained as a result of a military disaster in the Italian port of Bari. Despite the fact that chemical warfare had been outlawed by international treaty after World War I, considerable stockpiles of mustard gas were held by the US. In 1943, they transferred a large shipment of mustard gas bombs to Italy by ship. While in the Adriatic port of Bari, the US Liberty Ship *SS John Harvey*, which was carrying around 60,000 kg of mustard gas, was attacked and sunk by the Luftwaffe and the gas was released killing and maiming many sailors and civilians. Autopsies carried out on the dead revealed marked changes in their white cell counts and in the regression of their lymphoid tissue. These findings further stimulated interest and research into mustard gas derivatives as potential chemotherapeutic agents.

Both the early patient studies in Yale and the Bari incident were classified and the first reports of the successful use of this treatment were not published until after World War II in 1946. (7)

But of all the drug discoveries that might be attributed to serendipity, perhaps the greatest took place not on a battlefield in the midst of war, but on the window-sill of a London teaching hospital in the 1920s.

The first antibiotic

On 3 September 1928, Alexander Fleming (fig. 6.2) returned to work from his summer holiday. He was then Professor of

Bacteriology at St Mary's Hospital, London and that Monday morning he began to review petri dishes containing cultures of Staphylococcus — bacteria that cause a range of infections in man. In one dish he noticed an unusual phenomenon. In addition to the small discrete bacterial colonies, there was a growth of mould, around which there was a halo free of bacteria. (9, 10)

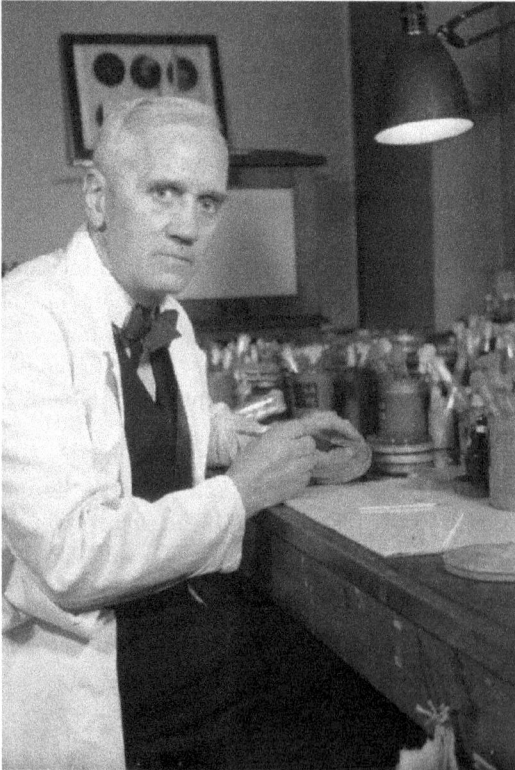

Figure 6.2. Alexander Fleming (1881-1955) in his laboratory at St Mary's Hospital, London. (Public Domain)

The mould would later be identified as *Penicillium notatum* and Fleming postulated that it had secreted something that had inhibited the bacterial growth. He initially described this as 'mould juice' and went on to discover that it would inhibit a wide range of other pathogenic bacteria including *Streptococcus*, *Menigococcus* and the bacteria responsible for diphtheria. Early attempts to isolate the inhibitory factor, which Fleming named penicillin, proved unsuccessful. Despite this, he published his initial findings in 1929, and although Fleming alludes to 'its possible use in bacterial infections' in his paper, he seems more interested in penicillin's potential as an analytical tool in the bacteriology laboratory. (9)

Fleming had doubtless accidentally contaminated his petri dishes, perhaps by leaving them by an open window. The *Penicillium* that found its way on to his plates might have come from mould spores from beer in the Fountains Abbey Ale House across the road from his lab in St. Mary's Hospital. At least, a hopeful plaque outside the pub in question claims Sir Alexander as 'a loyal regular' and takes credit for its part in the discovery of penicillin in 1928. Whatever the source, this was a mistake that when understood led to the advent of the antibiotic era.

Penicillin may have remained little more than a curious laboratory finding had it not been for the work of others, most notably the team in Oxford led by Howard Florey and Ernst Chain. In 1939, they began their work on the isolation and purification of penicillin. (9, 10) As war broke out, the Oxford team were starved of resources, but not resourcefulness. Florey and Chain resorted to using a variety of recycled culture flasks. In Oxford's History of Science Museum you can still see an old sheep dip can, an enamel bed pan and even a three-tired contraption made from old metal biscuit tins that were used in their early experiments. (fig. 6.3) Soon, the Oxford laboratory was turned into a penicillin factory.

In 1940, the Oxford team completed a series of critically important animal studies, showing that mice treated with penicillin could be protected from *Streptococcus* infection (11). The first human study took place the following year in 1941, when a 43-year old man who was suffering from a life-threatening infection became the first to be treated with the Oxford penicillin. Initially, he made a good recovery, but as supplies of the precious drug ran out he relapsed and died. (10)

Further clinical trials were more successful and quickly it was decided to make the production of penicillin a priority. Because of the lack of resources in wartime Britain and the need for further specialised input, the project was shifted to the US and to a major collaboration involving a number of drug companies and academic groups. This work was fraught with difficulty and the challenges of the scale-up process were summarised by Pfizer's John L. Smith when he said, 'The mould is as temperamental as an opera singer, the yields are low, the isolation is difficult, the extraction is murder, the purification invites disaster, and the assay is unsatisfactory.' (Quoted in 10)

However, the difficulties were met and overcome, and large-scale production of penicillin was achieved in time for the D-day landings in 1944. The drug became widely available to the public shortly thereafter.

The American Chemical Society and the Royal Society of Chemistry have since designated the development of penicillin as an 'International Historic Chemical Landmark' and Fleming, Chain and Florey were jointly awarded the 1945 Nobel Prize in Medicine or Physiology for their work. (10)

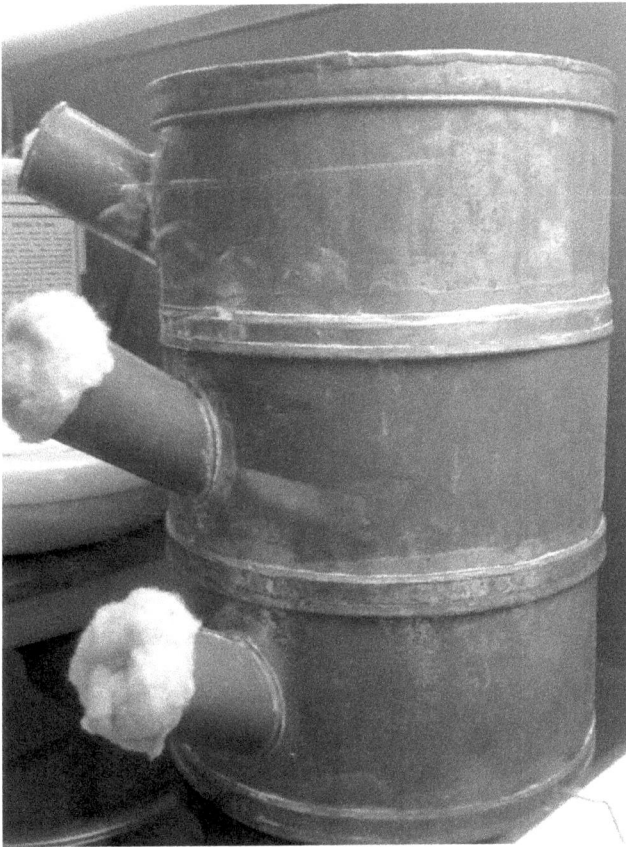

Figure 6.3. Penicillin culture vessel made from three tiered biscuit tins used by the Oxford Research group in the 1940s on display in the Museum of the History of Science, Oxford. (Photo by the author)

Despite the fact the Fleming is hailed as the discoverer of penicillin, he was not directly involved in the development of the drug and it is easy to diminish his role. Let us not forget, however, that Fleming had already been lauded for his work on the discovery of lysozyme — the antibacterial enzyme found in human tears. He was already well-acquainted with the concept of chemical inhibition of bacterial growth when he stumbled upon the *Penicillium* mould on his petri dishes. As that other great microbiologist Louis Pasteur had said many years before, 'Chance favours the mind that is well-prepared.' And Fleming was prepared. Had he simply discarded his contaminated plates without pausing to examine the halos of inhibited bacterial growth around the mould, and if he had not asked why such a thing had happened, we would not have penicillin.

Re-purposing

The unexpected can also play a role in the successful discovery of new drugs. As any new compound is carefully evaluated it may become clear that the drug, while having some of the specified effects under test, may also possess other qualities. Such unexpected events may redirect the development of a drug mid-stream and allow for the discovery of important new treatments. One of the most obvious example of this took place only twenty years ago.

In the early 1990s, a team working in Pfizer's research laboratories in England were investigating selective blockers of a phosphodiesterase called PDE5, which they believed may have a role in vasoconstriction. (12) By developing a powerful and selective inhibitor of this enzyme, they hoped to produce a new treatment for angina pectoris, which is characterized by narrowing of the coronary arteries that supply blood and oxygen to the heart muscle. Early work with the most promising candidate, known at the time as UK-92480, showed that it did indeed cause some vasodilatation in healthy volunteers, but it was short-acting and often caused muscle aches. Despite these disappointing results, in one early study, male volunteers also reported an unexpected side effect — that of increased erections a few days after the initial test dose. In further studies investigating the pharmacology of the new enzyme inhibitor, still as a potential anti-angina drug, increased erections were being further reported and the research team decided it might be time to look into this as a potentially new indication for the drug.

After successful pilot trials against placebos in patients with erectile dysfunction, larger studies were conducted in the UK, France and Sweden followed by much larger longer-term clinical trials world-wide.

The project that had first set out to find an inhibitor of PDE5 had begun in 1986. Four years later UK-92480 was selected as a candidate to enter clinical development for cardiovascular indications, but these ground to a halt after disappointing results. The first pilot studies in erectile dysfunction were completed in 1993. After another four years of research Pfizer had a sufficiently complete dossier of data that they applied for a license from the regulatory authorities in 1997, and UK-92480, now called sildenafil citrate, was approved as Viagra by the FDA as the first oral treatment for erectile dysfunction. (13) The drug became the fastest selling drug in history and was prescribed for over 30 million men world-wide.

But the story does not end there, for further research on sildenafil revealed it to be a candidate for the treatment of another condition. Between 2000-2002 there were a number of reports in the literature of patients whose pulmonary hypertension had been successfully treated with oral sildenafil. This prompted further clinical trials, and in 2005 sildenafil was approved as Revatio for the treatment of pulmonary arterial hypertension by the FDA and the EMEA (13).

The leader of the Pfizer research team Ian Osterloh said in one interview, 'It's immensely rewarding to know our work has benefited so many people. It is this fact that makes the long days and frustration, which are part and parcel of the development of pharmaceuticals, bearable'. And in acknowledgement of the collaborative efforts that are essential to modern drug development he added, 'I remind myself that I was just one member of a large team — experts in about 100 disciplines played a part in making Viagra available to patients.' (12)

Drug hunting

While luck has undoubtedly played a part in drug discovery, hard work and innovation have also been the weapons of those in search of new medicines. As our understanding of the workings of the cell has developed alongside our expertise in organic chemistry and pharmacology, new possibilities have opened up for a more rational approach to drug discovery. Armed with new knowledge and equipped with new techniques, the 20th century would become the era of the drug-hunters. Before the hunt could begin, however, some essential groundwork needed to be done.

Receptor Theory

In the last quarter of the 19th century, physiologists and pharmacologists were struggling with a basic problem — how did chemicals interact with tissues and cells?

A variety of answers were explored. Did they exert their actions by stimulating or inhibiting the nerve fibres that permeated such tissues; did they passively enter cells and exert their actions directly on some aspect of the cell's internal machinery; could they bind to some specific elements either in the cell or on its surface and indirectly effect their actions in this way?

The latter solution is what we now know as the 'receptor theory' and it has become central to our modern understanding of cell biology and molecular pharmacology, but in the late 19th century it was very far from clear that this was the answer.

What would become the receptor theory has two founding fathers who approached the same scientific question from entirely different angles. Their work was complimentary and ultimately consistent but was almost certainly intellectually independent of each other.

Paul Ehrlich, whom we met at the beginning of this chapter, was a bacteriologist and immunologist working in Berlin and he was primarily interested in the interaction of toxins and anti-toxins on cells. (14) (fig. 6.4) John Newport Langley, working in Cambridge, was a physiologist trying to understand how compounds such as pilocarpine, nicotine and extracts of the adrenal glands interacted and caused pharmacological effects on tissues such as smooth muscle and the salivary glands. (15) (fig. 6.5)

Although Ehrlich initially referred to his hypothetical binding structures on cells as 'side chains' he did coin the term 'receptor' in 1900, when he wrote:

> For the sake of brevity, that combining group of the protoplasmic molecule to which the introduced group is anchored will hereafter be termed "receptor". (16)

Langley referred to his hypothetical cellular components as 'receptive substances' and despite being aware of Ehrlich's terminology persisted in his use of this more ambiguous and less obviously structural term. Langley, unlike Ehrlich, viewed his 'receptive substances' as having a key role in the actions of drugs. Only later, would Ehrlich see that his receptors might have a role in pharmacology.

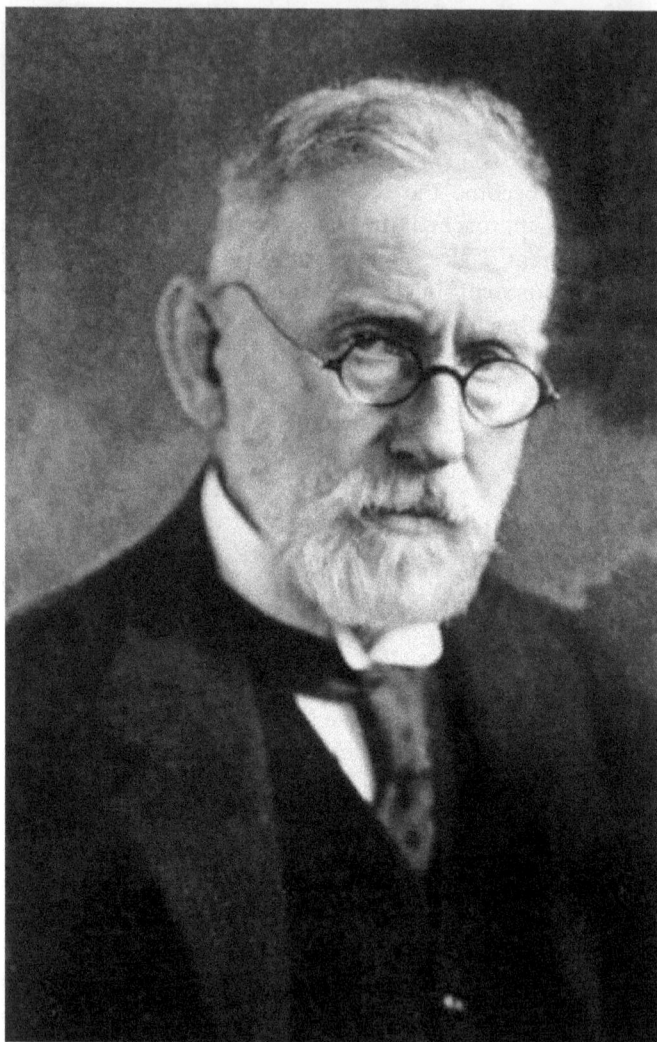

Figure 6.4. Paul Ehrlich (1854-1915) (Wellcome Library, London. Wellcome Images)

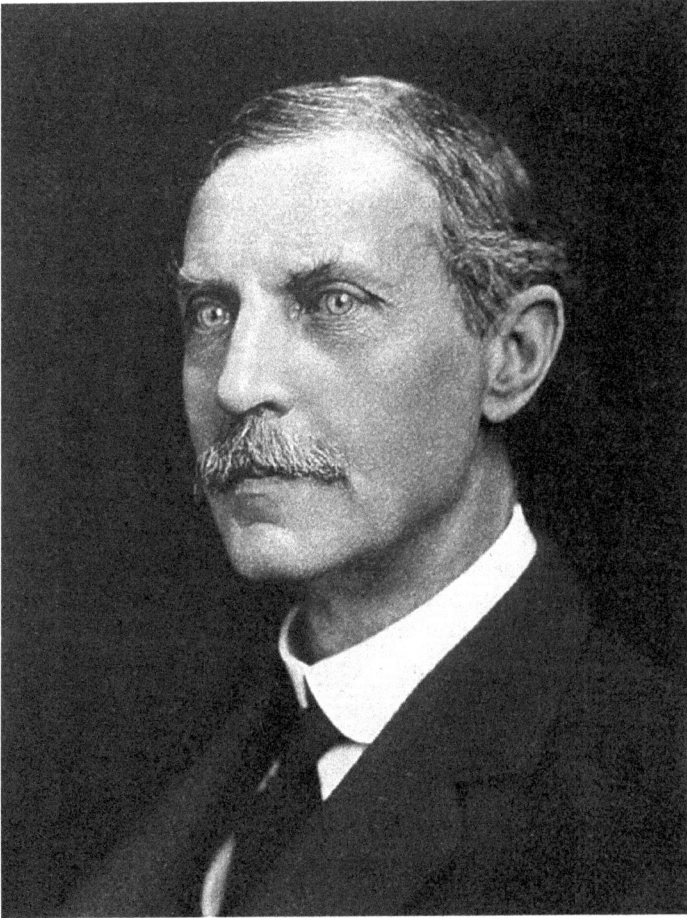

Figure 6.5. John Newport Langley (1852-1925)
(Wellcome Library, London. Wellcome Images)

The nascent receptor theory took a foothold in the early years of the 20th century, but it would be several decades before it would be widely accepted. And indeed it would take until the 1960s before the theory would have its first major impact on the discovery and development of new drugs.

If Ehrlich and Langley were the fathers of receptor theory, it has also had several godparents who facilitated its path from theory to accepted mechanistic explanation of drug-cell interactions. Chief amongst these was the pharmacologist Alfred Joseph Clark. Working in London and Edinburgh on the neurotransmitter acetylcholine, Clark performed detailed quantitative experiments that supported and extended the receptor theory. In particular, his mathematical approach in the 1920s and 30s demonstrated that the pharmacological action of a drug would be 'directly proportional to the number of receptors occupied'. (Quoted in 17). This work was crucial to the acceptance of the receptor theory and one historian argues that it was largely through Clark's work that the theory found acceptance in pharmacology (18). However, for the theory to find an application took another step and that was provided by the work of the American pharmacologist Raymond P. Ahlquist.

In 1948, Ahlquist offered a refinement in our understanding of the physiology of the adrenergic receptors by drawing a distinction between alpha- and beta-adrenoceptors. (19) This work, although published, lay relatively unrecognised and unacknowledged in the scientific literature for a decade before it was read by James Black, a young Scottish research scientist who had recently started work with the British drug company ICI (20). Black would become one of the most renowned of the 20th century drug-hunters and his discoveries would transform medical practice and ultimately 30 years later earn him the Nobel Prize in Medicine or Physiology. (fig. 6.6)

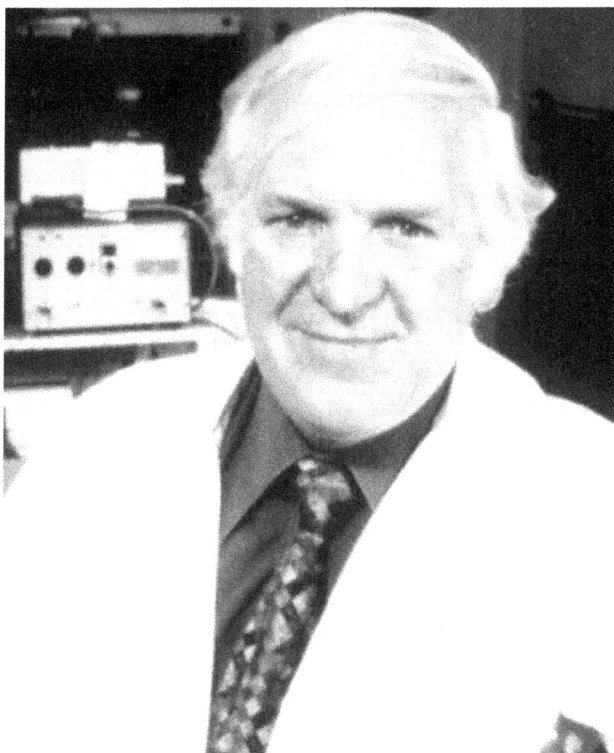

Figure 6.6. Sir James Black (1924-2010) (Public Domain)

Receptor blockade

The pharmaceutical company Eli Lilley had synthesised an analogue of the drug isoprenaline, called dichloroisoproterenol or DCI. After further research on this new compound they had designated it as a 'beta-adrenergic blocking drug', a term that would later be cropped to 'beta-blocker' (21).

Black realised this finding vindicated Ahlquist's dual receptor theory and recognised that DCI could be the starting point of his search at ICI for a clinically useful beta-blocker. The ICI team altered the structure of DCI and first came up with pronethalol in 1960, a beta-blocker that would be launched in 1963 as Alderlin, but which would later be withdrawn because of its carcinogenicity in animal models.

Despite the launch of Alderlin, Black was sure that a better version could be developed and by November 1962 a further 269 compounds had been synthesised. The synthesis of these allied compounds took place not only as part of Black's search for a superior beta-blocker, but also for sound commercial reasons — to protect ICI's patent and to ensure a similar compound could not be introduced into the market by a competitor (20). Black was looking for a beta-blocker that would be longer acting, have greater resistance to catecholamine 'breakthrough' and show less penetration of the central nervous system. He did not find his perfect drug, but amongst the candidates Black did discover No. 45,520, which had 10-20 times greater activity than pronethalol and a better therapeutic ratio in man between the doses that were blocking and toxic. This drug was propranolol. Licensed in 1965 and marketed by ICI as Inderal, this beta-blocker was initially indicated for angina and subsequently for hypertension, and became one of the most successful drugs of all time.

Receptor theory would be further exploited by Black in the field of gastroenterology, with his discovery of the H_2-receptor antagonist cimetidine, and by others in the development of new drugs in respiratory medicine, obstetrics, endocrinology and psychiatry. The 1960s and 70s have indeed been called 'the age of the receptor' (22), and it was Black's discovery of propranolol that did much to give the receptor theory a practical application in pharmacology.

Design and engineering of new drugs

Shortly before he won his Nobel Prize, James Black, in a lecture to the UK Pharmaceutical Marketing Society, said, 'The most fruitful basis of the discovery of a new drug is to start with an old drug.' (23)   There is much to commend this approach: Black developed propranolol from isoprenaline; and we saw earlier in Chapter 5 how Hoffmann developed Aspirin from salicylic acid and Heroin from morphine.   But, this approach is not the only way to develop a new drug, especially as our understanding of biochemistry and molecular pharmacology advances.   For example, could we study the exact structure of our defined molecular target and engineer a molecule that would fit?

The first example where this approach was used successfully was in the development of a topical treatment for the disease glaucoma.   This condition is caused by raised pressure within the eye and it is treated by strategies to reduce that pressure. Traditionally, this has been done using inhibitors of carbonic anhydrase, the enzyme that catalyses a key step in the secretion of aqueous humour in the anterior and posterior chambers of the eye.   Although systemic carbonic anhydrase inhibitors work, they cause significant side effects, so a topical alternative was sought. (24)

By studying the three-dimensional structure of the conical binding cavity in carbonic anhydrase II (the isoenzyme found within the secretory cells) researchers at Merck were able to develop a basic prototype compound. (25) This molecule could then be further modified by chemical subgroup substitution to improve the fit with the target enzyme, in much the same way as a tailor might take an off-the-peg jacket and through alterations make it truly bespoke.

The resulting tailor-made drug was Dorzolamide and this was approved for use as a topical treatment for glaucoma in 1995. This drug was the first human therapy to be developed through a strategy of structure-based design. (26)

In order for this strategy to become a reality, we need access to high-resolution three-dimensional structural information that will provide us with data at an atomic level. These data will be obtained through such techniques as X-Ray crystallography and NMR spectroscopy. When we combine these forms of imaging with sophisticated computer-aided molecular design we then have the possibility of *de novo* drug design.

Other drugs have been invented in this way since Dorzolamide, and many more are likely to be in the future, but this approach might only be fruitful if the clinical problem in question can be associated with a single receptor function, such as a specific enzyme or transport protein. Many diseases, however, are unfortunately multi-factorial and such an approach may prove less than successful in every case.

Revisiting magic bullets

We began with Paul Ehrlich's quest for his 'magic bullet' at the beginning of the 20th century and although we have come a long way it seems appropriate to end there too.

Ehrlichs's search stemmed from his early work on developing staining techniques for different bacteria. If a chemical in the form of a dye could be taken up specifically by an organism, might it not be possible to find a chemical or dye with a similarly specific affinity that would also be selectively toxic to the bacterium? (14)   This was the question that exercised Ehrlich and his team.

The search began as early as 1891, when he experimented with the clinical use of the dye methylene blue, successfully treating patients with malaria. In 1904, he and his colleagues had further limited success with the dye trypan red in animal models of trypanosomiasis. Next, Ehrlich turned to organic arsenic containing compounds, which would eventually yield his first major success. Using aminophenyl arsenic acid, which had been marketed as a treatment for African sleeping sickness, as a starting point, Ehrlich's team synthesised a series of analogues over the next few years.

With the discovery in 1905 of the causative agent of syphilis, the spirochaete *Treponema pallidum*, Ehrlich was encouraged by colleagues to re-evaluate his series of arsenical compounds as a treatment for this disease. (27)

This work was made possible by the arrival in Ehrlich's lab of Sahachiro Hata, a Japanese student who had developed a rabbit model of syphilis. In the experiments that followed, compound No. 606, arsphenamine, proved to be highly effective. After further testing, human clinical trials were performed. The success of these prompted the German drug company Hoechst to market the drug as Salvarsan, meaning the arsenic that saves. (27)

This was the first truly effective treatment for syphilis and it would continue to be used in a variety of formulations for the next 30 years. Although hailed as Ehrlich's long sought 'magic bullet', Salvarsan was not quite as charmed as he might have wished. The drug, although effective, was associated with significant and unpleasant side effects.

Since that time the hunt for magic bullets has continued not only in infectious diseases, but also in cancer, cardiovascular disease, psychiatry, and every other clinical field. To find the drug that effectively does the job we want it to do and nothing else remains the holy grail of modern pharmacology and the search for the truly 'magic' bullet continues to this day.

Conclusions

As we study the discovery of new drugs, we are confronted with a remarkable array of possibilities. In particular, over the decades of the 20th century, scientists and clinicians across the world have used every conceivable approach to seek out new treatments.

In some cases, drugs have apparently landed in our laps. Such happy accidents can lead to discovery, but they are only fortunate if the insights they offer are noticed and acted upon by scientists. Every day in every lab and every clinic in the world, serendipity holds out its hand and offers us new knowledge. But we need the wit to realise it and those who do are exceptional. The physiologist Albert Szent-Gyorgi, who won the 1937 Nobel Prize in Medicine or Physiology for his work on Vitamin C and the citric acid cycle, realised this. He said, 'Discovery consists in seeing what everyone else has seen and thinking what no one else has thought.' It is this simple attribute that separates the great scientists from the run of the mill — that allows paradigm changing discoveries to be made based on the simplest of observations in those experiments designed for us by serendipity.

But good luck will only take us so far. We also need the creative minds of scientists such as Ehrlich, Langley, Chain, Florey and Black, who have the ability to make new connections between apparently disparate facts and, through careful observation and study, unwrap the truth.

And more and more, we are seeing the power of truly multi-disciplinary approaches to drug discovery — pharmacologists working with computer scientists; physicians working with physicists; and organic chemists working with mathematicians. Drug discovery is no less a challenge in the 21st century than it was in the past, but today we are better equipped than ever to meet it.

References

1.   Ehrlich P. Experimental researches on specific therapy. On immunity with special relationship between distribution and action of antigens. *Harben Lecture* 1908 Lewis, London, p 107.

2.   Williams KJ. The introduction of 'chemotherapy' using arsphenamine – the first magic bullet. *James Lind Library Bulletin: Commentaries on the history of treatment evaluation* 2009. http://www.jameslindlibrary.org/articles/the-introduction-of-chemotherapy-using-arsphenamine-the-first-magic-bullet/ (Accessed 8 January 2016)

3.   Donaldson IML. Ambroise Paré's accounts of new methods for treating gunshot wounds and burns. *James Lind Library Bulletin: Commentaries on the history of treatment evaluation* 2004. http://www.jameslindlibrary.org/articles/ambroise-pares-accounts-of-new-methods-for-treating-gunshot-wounds-and-burns/ (Accessed 8 January 2016).

4.   Paré A. *La Méthode de traicter les playes faictes par hacquebutes et aultres bastons à feu et de celles qui sont faictes par flèches, dardz et semblables, aussy des combustions spécialement faictes par la pouldre à canon, composée par Ambroyse Paré.* V. Gaulterot, Paris, 1545 fol. 52 v.

5.   Fitzgerald GJ. Chemical warfare and medical response during World War I. *American Journal of Public Health* 2008; 98: 611-25.

6.   Krumbhaar EB. Role of the blood and the bone marrow in certain forms of gas poisoning. *Journal of the American Medical Association* 1919; 72: 39-41.

7.   Fenn JE, Udelsman R.   First use of intravenous chemotherapy cancer treatment: rectifying the record. *Journal of the American College of Surgeons* 2011; 212: 413-7.

8.   Goodman LS, Wintrobe MM, Dameshek W, Goodman MJ, Gilman A, McLennan MT. Nitrogen mustard therapy. Use of methyl-bis(beta-chloroethyl)amine hydrochloride and tris(beta-chloroethyl)amine hydrochloride for Hodgkin's disease, lymphosarcoma, leukemia and certain allied and miscellaneous disorders. *Journal of the American Medical Association* 1946; 132: 126-32.

9.   Fleming A.   On the bacterial action of cultures of a Pencillium, with special reference to their use in the isolation of *B. influenzae*.   *British Journal of Experimental Pathology* 1929; 10: 226-36.

10.   Aldridge S, Parascandola J, Sturchio JL. *The discovery and development of penicillin 1928-1945*. Alexander Fleming Museum, London, 1999. http://www.acs.org/content/dam/acsorg/education/whati schemistry/landmarks/flemingpenicillin/the-discovery-and-development-of-penicillin-commemorative-booklet.pdf (Accessed 8 January 2016).

11.   Chain E, Florey HW, Gardner AD, Heatley NG, Jennings MA, Orr-Ewing J, Sanders AG.   Penicillin as a chemotherapeutic agent. *Lancet* 1940; ii: 226-8.

12.   Osterloh I. How I discovered Viagra   *Cosmos* July, 2007. https://cosmosmagazine.com/life-sciences/how-i-discovered-viagra (Accessed 8 January 2016).

13.   Ghofrani HA, Osterloh IH, Grimminger F. Sildenafil: from

angina to erectile dysfunction to pulmonary hypertension and beyond. *Nature Reviews Drug Discovery* 2006; 5: 689-702.

14.   Prüll C-R. Part of a scientific master plan? Paul Ehrlich and the origins of his receptor concept. *Medical History* 2003; 47: 332-56.

15.   Maehle A-H. "Receptive substances": John Newport Langley (1852-1925) and his path to a receptor theory of drug action. *Medical History* 2004; 48: 153-74.

16.   Ehrlich P, Morgenroth J. Über Haemolysine. Dritte Mittheilung. Berliner Klinische Wochenschrift 1900. In: Himmelweit F. (ed) *The Collected Papers of Paul Ehrlich in Four Volumes Vol 2. Immunology and Cancer Research* Pergamon Press, London, 1956-60. pp 205-12.

17.   Maehle A-H, Prüll C-R, Halliwell RF. The emergence of the drug receptor theory. *Nature Reviews* 2002; 1: 637-41.

18.   Parascandola J. A. J. Clark: quantitative pharmacology and the receptor theory. *Trends in Pharmacological Sciences* 1982; 3: 421-3.

19.   Ahlquist RP. A study of the adrenotropic receptors. *American Journal of Physiology* 1948; 153: 586-600.

20.   Quirke V. Putting theory into practice: James Black, receptor theory and the development of the beta-blockers at ICI, 1958-1978. *Medical History* 2006; 50: 69-92.

21.   Moran NC, Perkins ME. Adrenergic blockade of the mammalian heart by a dichloro analogue of isoproterenol. *Journal of Pharmacology and Experimental Therapeutics* 1958; 124: 223-37.

22.   Cuthbert AW. Men, molecules and machines. *Trends in Pharmacological Sciences* 1979; 1: 1-3.

23. Connor S, Charles D, Kingman S, Lesser F. Drug pioneers win Nobel laureate. *New Scientist* 1988; 22 October: 26-7.

24. Talele TT, Khedkar SA, Rigby AC. Successful applications of computer aided drug discovery: moving drugs from concept to the clinic. *Current Topics in Medicinal Chemistry* 2010; 10: 127-41.

25. Greer J, Erickson JW, Baldwin JJ, Varney MD. Application of the three-dimensional structures of protein target molecules in structure-based drug design. *Journal of Medicinal Chemistry* 1994; 37: 1035-54.

26. Timmerman H, Gubernator K, Böhm HJ, Mannhold R, Kubinyi H. *Structure-based Ligand Design (Methods and Principles in Medicinal Chemistry)*. Wiley-VCH, Weinheim, 1998.

27. Bosch F, Rosich L. The contributions of Paul Ehrlich to pharmacology: a tribute on the occasion of the centenary of his Nobel Prize. *Pharmacology* 2008; 82: 171-9.

——— ∎ ———

7

The Medico-industrial Complex

The Beginnings of the Pharmaceutical Industry

Introduction

Any history of drug research, no matter how brief, would be seriously lacking if it did not look at the role of the developing pharmaceutical industry. This industry, which is now a multi-national, multi-billion dollar enterprise, has been intimately involved in the discovery, development and testing of new drugs for many years. Just how many years is debatable, for to look at this aspect of the history of our subject we need to define what exactly we mean by the pharmaceutical industry.

When you look for histories of the pharmaceutical industry there are two surprises. First, very few detailed histories have been written. This is unexpected because the pharmaceutical industry is one of the largest on Earth, touching almost everyone in one way or another. The second surprise is that in those scant histories that do exist, the birth date of the pharmaceutical industry is usually given as the mid-19th century, with the founding of the German drug company E. Merck.

Now, for as long as there have been people I suspect there have been men and women making drugs and remedies and probably selling them — if not for money, at least in exchange for something of equal value. Indeed, we have seen in the previous chapters that there has been a very long interest in therapeutics. Over many centuries there has been the compounding of herbs and chemicals to create medicines; there have been concerns over quality of drugs, their safety and effectiveness; there has been protectionism and there has even been bulk production.

Perhaps all the hallmarks of a modern pharmaceutical industry have been in place — in some cases for centuries — so what exactly do we mean when we say that the first pharmaceutical company was established in the mid-19th century? Why do we choose that moment to mark the birth of a new industry?

The Pharmaceutical Industry

The primary hallmark of the pharmaceutical industry is surely the mass production of drugs. Closely related to this industrialization of scale, however, are the needs for quality control, mass marketing and sales and, in order for a company to grow, research and development and a global outlook. On top of this, a need for protectionism will inevitably evolve alongside the development of new business models appropriate for the time and the place.

If mass production alone were the only characteristic of industry, then perhaps we should date the birth of the pharmaceutical industry to the time of batch preparation of theriac in the 16th century. Or perhaps the honour should go to the French chemists Pelletier and Caventou who in 1826 extracted 1,800 kg of quinine sulphate from 150 tons of imported cinchona bark and in some historians' opinion started the pharmaceutical industry. (1)

However, the drug company E. Merck does have a fair claim to be the oldest continuous pharmacy and pharmaceutical company in the world with its origins going back to an apothecary shop in Darmstadt, Germany in 1668. (2, 3). Emanuel Merck (1794-1855), whose name lives on in several of the pharmaceutical giants of the 21st century, took over the Engel-Apotheke in 1816, which had been run by six previous generations of his family, and transformed it into a bulk manufacturer of alkaloids and other medicinal products (figs 7.1 & 7.2). In 1850, he created the company E. Merck. (3) Merck had certainly built a reputation for quality even before his decision to incorporate, as evidenced by the endorsement he received in 1849 from Karl Friedrich Mohr, a professor of pharmacy in Berlin, who wrote the following in 'Comments on Prussian Pharmacopeia',

> I would prefer to take morphine from Merck than from an unknown manufacturer. Just as nobody is prevented from manufacturing permitted medicines, I don't want to see pharmacists being obliged to make medicines with which they have no experience. This is the case for morphine. (3)

The industrialization of pharmaceuticals had truly begun and this model would soon be copied across the country and the world.

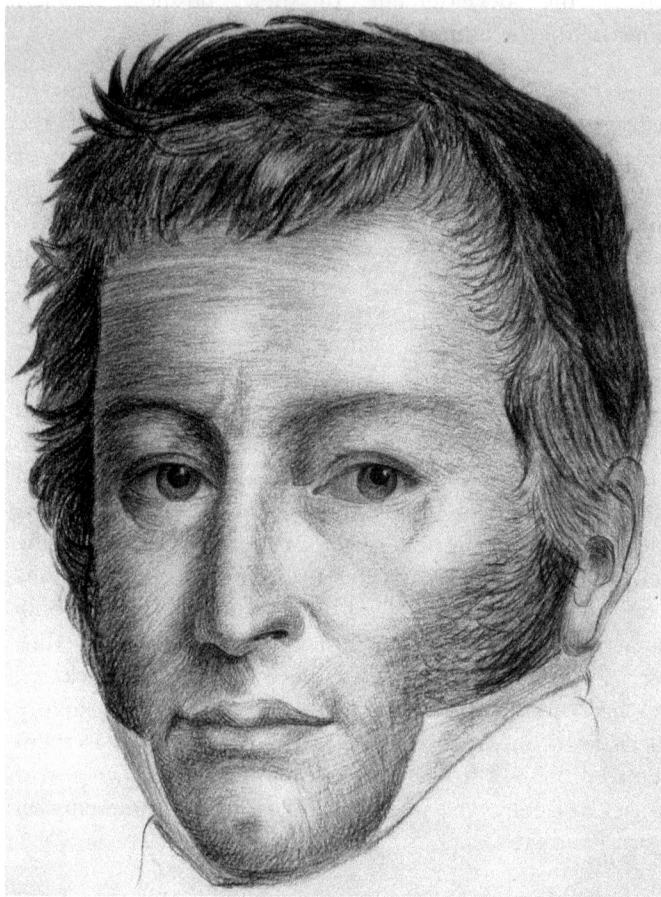

Figure 7.1. Emanuel Merck (1794-1855) (Used with permission, © Merck KGaA, Darmstadt Germany)

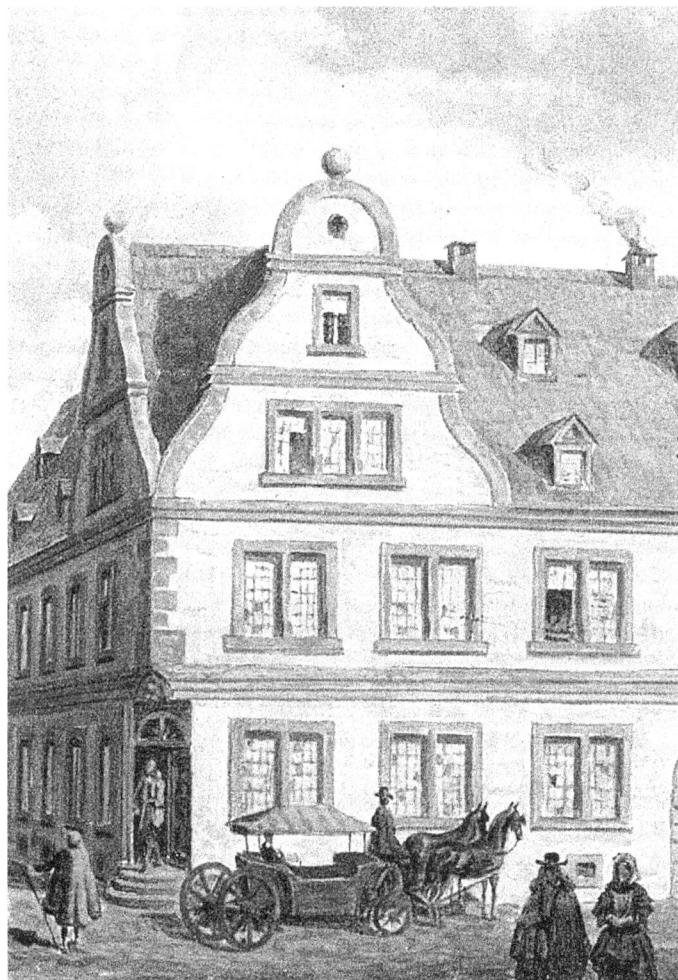

Figure 7.2. The Engel-Apotheke, Darmstadt
(Used with permission, © Merck KGaA, Darmstadt Germany)

The German pharmaceutical industry

A number of the major drug companies that developed, especially in Germany, did not, however, have pharmacy backgrounds. Instead, their expertise lay in chemistry. The German dye industry had been flourishing and due to complex patent protection these highly sought after commodities generated large profits for a group of German companies including Bayer, Hoechst and BASF.

The practicalities of chemical synthesis that were employed to manufacture synthetic dyes were the same ones that could be used to produce drugs. In the dye industry, the people, the plant and the processes were all in place; all that was needed was the incentive to diversify.

This incentive came in the mid-1880s with changes in the pricing convention for red dyes and the rising costs of raw materials that put financial pressures on the large chemical and dyestuff manufactures. (4) As the dye companies shifted their industrial laboratories to the manufacture of drugs and entered the pharmaceutical market they became major competitors for more traditional pharmacy-based companies such as Merck.

What these chemical and dye houses also had was a corporate structure that included different specialized divisions including manufacturing, sales and marketing and quality control. This structure would provide the model for much of the pharmaceutical industry in the next century.

Patent protection

Another hallmark of the modern pharmaceutical industry is the protection of patent rights and it is useful to look at this in the context of its impact on drug research.

While patent protection may be seen as a major incentive to develop and manufacture newer, better drugs because of the assurance of a return on any investment, the patenting of drugs is a relatively new phenomenon. In the 19th century, with the notable exception of the United States, all European countries excluded drugs from the inventions that could be protected by means of intellectual property rights. (5) It has been argued that this was neither due to an oversight nor was it due to disinterest, but rather it was the result of heated debate and controversial decisions at the highest political level. (5) Up to World War II, this was largely the situation with the central argument being whether it was 'patents for profits' or 'patents for quality control'. (6, 7) After the war, there was a rapidly expanding industry and powerful lobbying for the patent protection that the major drug companies saw as essential for their continued existence. As a result, most countries enacted legislation that would protect newly developed drugs.

While drugs themselves were not the subject of patents in Europe for most of the century, after 1850 many manufacturers sought to protect the chemical processes used in the synthesis of their new drugs and these were regularly patented. Drug names would also be trademarked as we have seen with Aspirin and Heroin.

Thus, the principles of protectionism that are inherent to any large organization were already embedded in the industry from its earliest days.

Research in the pharmaceutical industry

While there is a very great deal that could be written about the development of the pharmaceutical industry, I want to focus here on the role played by this developing industry in drug research.
The early role of the pharmaceutical industry in research has already been touched on in previous chapters. In chapter 5, we

visited the laboratories of the German drug company Bayer in the late 19th century to witness the development of new drugs. In chapter 6, we saw how industry played a key role in the development and commercialization of drugs such as penicillin, propranolol and sildenafil.

Thus, we have seen some of the impact of the early pharmaceutical industry on drug research, but it is probably useful to focus on how this industry has developed in the post-World War II era to understand its present position and significance.

From its beginnings in the German dyestuff industry, through a growing understanding of organic chemistry and pharmacology, the pharmaceutical industry in 1945 was primed to become an increasingly research aware and research oriented endeavour.

From 1945 to the 1980s the dominant organizational structure to be found in the industry was that of a vertically integrated, multi-national company (8). This consisted of in-house research and development laboratories, manufacturing facilities and marketing and sales divisions. This was a direct legacy of the chemical and dye industry models from Germany in the 1880s.

Pharmaceutical companies in this era would finance their research from their own funds and would incur relatively little debt (9, 10). According to one economist, 'This was viewed as a strategic response to the risks involved in developing new pharmaceuticals — in particular, long investment periods, high costs, and variable outcomes.' (8)

At that time, the actual work of drug discovery was mainly by means of large-scale random screening of compound libraries to see if any relevant and commercially exploitable biological effect could be uncovered. In some ways, this was a mechanized and methodical approach seeking to emulate the natural serendipity that had furnished a number of previously very successful drugs. Where other researchers had stumbled upon new drugs, these companies were hoping that they too would chance upon a winner. They were, however, stacking the odds in their favour by studying not just one or two drugs but by systematically testing hundreds, if not thousands, of chemical entities.

This approach was successful and yielded a number of important new drug classes, such as broad spectrum antibiotics, corticosteroids, diuretics and antidepressants.

The development of these drugs was, however, becoming increasingly expensive and time consuming. When corrected for inflation the research costs per new drug brought to market have increased six-fold between the 1970s and the late 1990s — from US$138 million to US$802 million (8). This is in part due to tighter regulation of new drug introductions with the average number of patients in clinical trials supporting a licensing application being approximately 2,000 in the 1970s rising to more than 5,000 in the 1990s. (11)

New drug approvals peaked in the mid to late 1990s. Since that time there has been a relatively fallow period, despite the fact that R&D expenditure has risen steadily. Why should this be?

As existing high earning drugs come off patent and are challenged by a growing generic market, the major pharmaceutical companies face a significant pipeline problem if they do not have further 'blockbuster' products to fill the gaps. A blockbuster is defined within the industry as a product that achieves sales of US$ 1 billion or more. (8) Unfortunately, of those new drugs coming to market, fewer and fewer are deemed likely to earn this label.

In many ways, the low hanging fruit of pharmaceuticals have already been picked and eaten. Common diseases with clearly defined therapeutic targets have already been exploited; what remains are more complex diseases with either unknown or complex multifactorial aetiologies, such as Alzheimer's Disease, a number of degenerative diseases of the elderly and several major cancers.

These challenges have in part been the driver for some of the major structural changes within the industry in the last 20 years, both horizontal and vertical. (8) Large scale mergers and acquisitions have led to a more consolidated industry structure, while there has been a deconstruction of the classic, internal structure in most companies leading to greater outsourcing and partnerships with smaller drug development and biotechnology companies rather than on relying wholly on in-house drug discovery and development.

Despite this, there is little evidence that the horizontal restructuring of the industry has had any significant impact on new drug development and research performance. (12) In contrast, the vertical restructuring does appear to have led to improvements. (8)

But pharmaceutical companies have rarely worked alone. In the early days of the industry, many of the innovations that led to commercially successful products were from outside. Indeed, before World War I, all of the top ten drugs sold by Merck were invented by either university or freelance researchers. (2) These included the haemostatic drug Stypticin invented by Freund in 1897 and the first barbiturate, Veronal, invented by Fischer and von Mering in 1903. A greater emphasis on in-house research and development was heralded by the creation of centralized research laboratories. The first of these were established by Bayer in 1891 and followed by Wellcome in 1896, Merck in 1898 and Dupont in 1903. (2)

In the twenty years after World War II, there was a large surge in the invention and commercialization of new drugs. In this period, the main strength of industry was in chemistry, while that of their academic partners was clinical. This fostered a close symbiotic relationship between industry and academia that promoted the development of Clinical Pharmacology as a sub-specialty. (13)

As research regulation and complexity increased, industry started to take a number of these previously outsourced roles in-house. They employed their own specialists in clinical pharmacology, trial design, statistics and regulatory affairs. These moves ultimately changed the relationship that clinical academics had with industry from one of partner to that of contractor (13).

During the last 50 years, academic departments have continued to work closely with industry partners in a variety of ways. For much of that time this has been a very productive arrangement because the relationship has been 'complementary rather than competitive'. (8) The available evidence supports this symbiosis. When the R&D Heads of various pharmaceutical companies were interviewed it was found that around half of all new drugs brought to market between 1986-94 received 'very substantial aid' or 'could not have been developed (without substantial delay) in the absence of recent academic research.' (14). That said, almost all of these new drugs did not owe their origins to academia but to industry, with 93% of the 284 new drugs approved in the US in 1990-99 coming from commercial research and development (11), emphasizing the increasingly limited role that academia has in drug discovery.

Whether this fruitful collaboration between industry and academia will continue remains to be seen. Changing agendas, particularly within modern universities and their increasingly protective views of intellectual property are likely to adversely affect these industry-academia partnerships. In addition, further changes to the model of drug discovery, with increasing reliance on smaller biotechnology companies as feeders, is likely to further disrupt the relationship.

Pharma Today

By 2014, the global pharmaceutical market was worth US$ 300 billion per annum with the expectation that this will rise to US$ 400 billion by 2017. (15) The ten largest pharmaceutical companies control over one third of this market with sales of over US$ 10 billion per annum each and profit margins of around 30%. Six of these top companies are based in the US while the others are in Europe. The companies are estimated to spend approximately one third of their sales revenues on marketing, which represents twice what they spend on research and development. (16)

The WHO says there is now, 'an inherent conflict of interest between the legitimate business goals of manufacturers and the social, medical and economic needs of providers and the public to select and use drugs in the most rational way.' (15) This, in truth, is a conflict that has always been there, and always will be, while we live in a capitalist society, but one that has been brought into sharper focus in recent years.

Pharmaceutical companies are large businesses and like any other company in recent years they have struggled to meet the expectations of their investors. They have, like other industries, restructured and relocated to minimize their taxation, but have done so at a time when the public is being made acutely aware of such avoidance strategies used by large multi-nationals. Added to this there have been a number of high profile cases where drug companies have been found to have serious ethical shortcomings and have appeared to place profits ahead of the interests of patients.

Indeed, between January 2009 and February 2014, eleven drug

companies were fined a total of more than US$13 billion because of a range of illegal activities that included allegations of fraudulent marketing activities and the failure to report adverse event data for their drugs. (17)

These revelations have led to a growing public mistrust of the pharmaceutical industry and its practices, to such an extent that in a 2013 poll it was placed almost on a par with the Tobacco and Financial Industries. (18) Big pharma thus has a serious reputational problem, but this is largely of its own making. (17) The re-building of that reputation will be long and difficult, but it will incorporate an ethical approach to business and a refocus on its main consumers — patients. From a research perspective, this will most easily be achieved by engaging in a meaningful dialogue with patient groups. This will allow the industry to direct its research into areas that attend to patient needs and their health priorities. In addition, by taking on research projects that are deemed high priority, but not necessarily high profit, the industry can reaffirm its key role in society. One example of this might be the search for new classes of antibiotics to replace those that are being rendered ineffective because of bacterial resistance.

Of relevance here are the words of George W. Merck, who in 1950 was the Head of Merck & Co, one of the largest and most successful of the US drug houses. He said,

> We try never to forget that medicine is for the people. It is not for the profits. The profits follow, and if we have remembered that, they have never failed to appear. The better we have remembered it, the larger they have been. (19)

Thus, thinking of patients first and profits second may not only be more in tune with how the public would like to see the pharmaceutical industry operate, it may also make better business sense.

Of course, the pharmaceutical industry is a business, with responsibilities to its stockholders. But, it is more than that — it is also the powerhouse that will drive drug research through the 21ˢᵗ century. Such research, if it addresses the significant causes of human suffering, could have enormous benefits for the population. However, if it is merely used to develop a range of freshly patented me-too drugs or a range of remedies for half-invented conditions then it could be seen as merely a vehicle to turn a profit, as well as a lost opportunity.

Conclusions

Without the pharmaceutical industry we would not have our modern formulary. Without the close collaborations that have existed over the last century between clinicians, scientists and industry, we would have nothing like the breadth of treatments that allow modern medicine to function. Without drug discovery, fuelled by energetic and innovative minds and occasionally helped along by the hand of chance, diseases would go untreated and suffering unrelieved.

We need drug discovery today just as we have always needed it. Even for the practice of medicine to stand still, we need to replace obsolete drugs and deal with those that no longer function effectively. For healthcare to advance, we need new therapeutic options for those diseases that have to date resisted treatment. We will always need better, safer drugs and our search for those 'magic bullets' should never end.

References

1.   Raviña E. *The Evolution of Drug Discovery: From Traditional Medicines to Modern Drugs.* Wiley-VCH, Weinheim, 2011.

2.   Burhop C. Pharmaceutical Research in Wilhelmine Germany: The Case of E. Merck. *Business History Review* 2009; 83: 475-503.

3.   Anon. *Merck from 1668 until today. Exploring new horizons.* Group Communications Merck, Darmstadt, 2013. http://merck.de/company.merck.de/de/images/Merck_Hist ory_EN_2013_tcm1613_105832.pdf?Version (Accessed 8 December 2014).

4.   Liebenau J. Ethical business: the formation of the pharmaceutical industry in Britain, Germany, and the United States before 1914. *Business History* 1988; 30: 116-29.

5.   Gaudillière J-P. How pharmaceuticals became patentable: the production and appropriation of drugs in the twentieth century. *History and Technology: An International Journal* 2008; 24: 99-106.

6.   American Medical Association. Conference on Medical Patents. *Journal of the American Association of Medicine* 1939; 113: 327-35.

7.   Anon. Manufacturers' point of view on medical patents in relation to public welfare. *Journal of the American Association of Medicine* 1939; 113: 419-27.

8.   Grabowski H. The evolution of the pharmaceutical industry over the past 50 years: A personal reflection. *International Journal of the Economics of Business* 2011; 18: 161-76.

9.   Grabowski H. The determinants of industrial research and development: a study of the chemical, drug, and petroleum industries. *Journal of Political Economy* 1968; 76: 292-306.

10.   Grabowski HG, Vernon JM. The determinants of R&D expenditures. In: Helms RB (Ed.), *Drugs and Health*, pp. 3-20 AEI, Washington, DC, 1981.

11.   DiMasi JA, Hansen RW, Grabowski HG. The price of innovation: new estimates of drug development costs. *Journal of Health Economics* 2003; 22: 151-85.

12.   Grabowski HG, Kyle MK. Mergers and alliances in

pharmaceuticals: effects on innovation and R&D productivity. In: Gugler K, Yurtogiv B (Eds), *The Economics of Corporate Governance and Mergers*, pp. 262-84, Edward Elgar, Northampton, 2008.

13.   Dollery CT. Clinical pharmacology – the first 75 years and a view of the future. *British Journal of Clinical Pharmacology* 2006; 61: 650-65.

14.   Mansfield E. Academic research and industrial innovation: an update of empirical findings. *Research Policy* 1998; 26: 773-6.

15.   WHO. Trade, foreign policy, diplomacy and health — Pharmaceutical Industry. 2014. http://www.who.int/trade/glossary/story073/en/ (Accessed 8 January 2016).

16.   Ferner R. A short history of pharmaceutical marketing *British Medical Journal* 2012; 345: e7801.

17.   Kessel M. Restoring the pharmaceutical industry's reputation. *Nature Biotechnology* 2014; 32: 983-90.

18.   Harris Interactive. *The Harris Poll 2013 RQ. Summary Report.* (Harris Interactive, Rochester, NY, February 2013) https://www.harrisinteractive.com/ vault/2013%20RQ%20Summary%20Report%20 FINAL.pdf (Accessed 7 October 2015).

19.   Merck GW. Speech at the Medical College of Virginia at Richmond. Quoted in New York Community Trust. 1950. http://www.nycommunitytrust.org/Portals/0/Uploads/Doc uments/BioBrochures/George%20W.%20Merck.pdf (Accessed 3 October 2015).

— ■ —

8

Born in Scandal

The Beginnings of Drug Regulation

Introduction

The American bioethicist Carol Levine noted that, 'the basic approach to the ethical conduct of research and approval of investigational drugs was born in scandal and reared in protectionism.' (1)

The scandals that have given birth to new drug legislation have become well-known, and they have been the subject of extensive debate and scholarship. (2) What is often less well known is the role played by one individual in the genesis of modern drug regulation. To be at the centre of one of the 20th century's drug scandals is remarkable enough; to be a key player in two is unprecedented. The star of both acts was a modest and unassuming woman called Frances Oldham Kelsey (fig. 8.1), who died in 2015 aged 101.

Kelsey was born in Canada in 1914, where she obtained her Bachelor and Masters degrees in pharmacology in 1934 and 1935. (3) At the height of the depression, with laboratory jobs difficult to come by, she decided to pursue graduate studies and at the suggestion of her professor at McGill she applied to Eugene Geiling, a distinguished researcher, who was establishing a new Department of Pharmacology in Chicago. (4) Kelsey's first brush with the kind of scandal that would shape modern drug legislation came in the second year of her doctoral studies at the University of Chicago, in 1937.

Sulfanilimide

The small American drug company S.E. Massengill Co. from Tennessee had decided to market the new drug sulfanilimide as an oral liquid preparation. This anti-bacterial in pill form had been highly effective in combatting infections, such as streptococcus, in the pre-antibiotic era. Thus, Massengill saw a market for it in children with throat and other infections — hence, their desire to offer it as a liquid preparation. The problems they faced, however, were that the drug was insoluble in water and quite unpalatable. The company's chief chemist and pharmacist, Harold Cole Watkins, experimented and was pleased to report that he had managed to dissolve the sulfanilimide in an ethanol-like solvent that even tasted sweet. As such, the drug would be sold as an 'elixir', or alcohol solution. However, the solvent was not alcohol, but diethylene glycol, the chief constituent of anti-freeze and highly toxic.

Pre-marketing safety testing was neither required by law nor contemplated by the company, and the 'elixir' was merely assessed for flavour, appearance and fragrance. After adding some pink colouring and raspberry flavouring, the company was satisfied on these counts and the preparation was mass-produced, bottled and shipped across the US in September 1937. (fig. 8.2) (4)

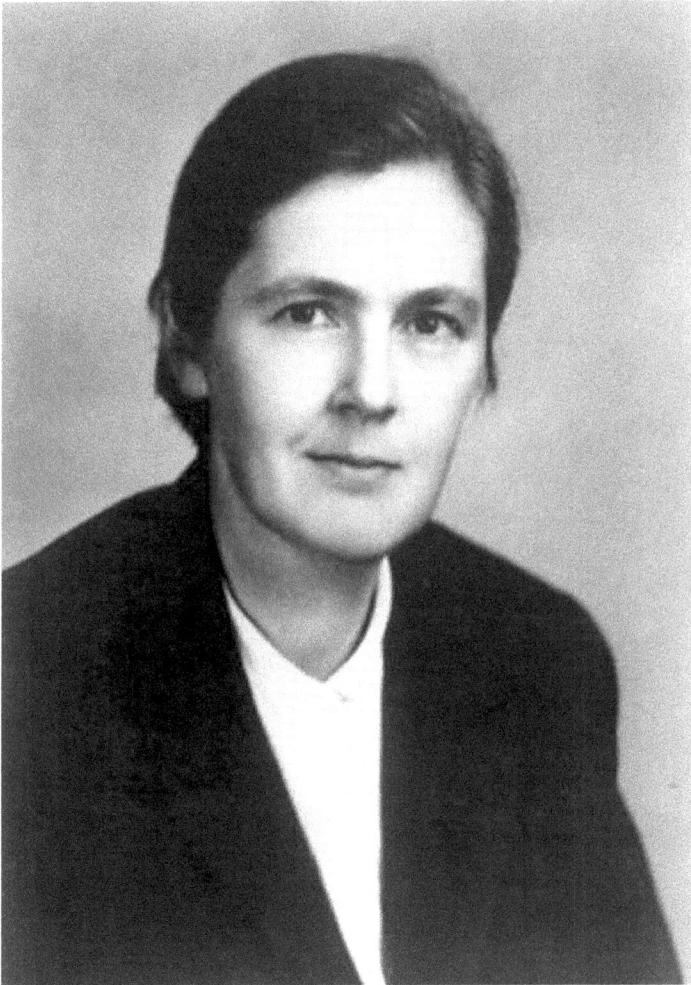

Figure 8.1. Frances Oldham Kelsey (1914-2015), photograph taken c1955. (Wikimedia commons: Public Domain)

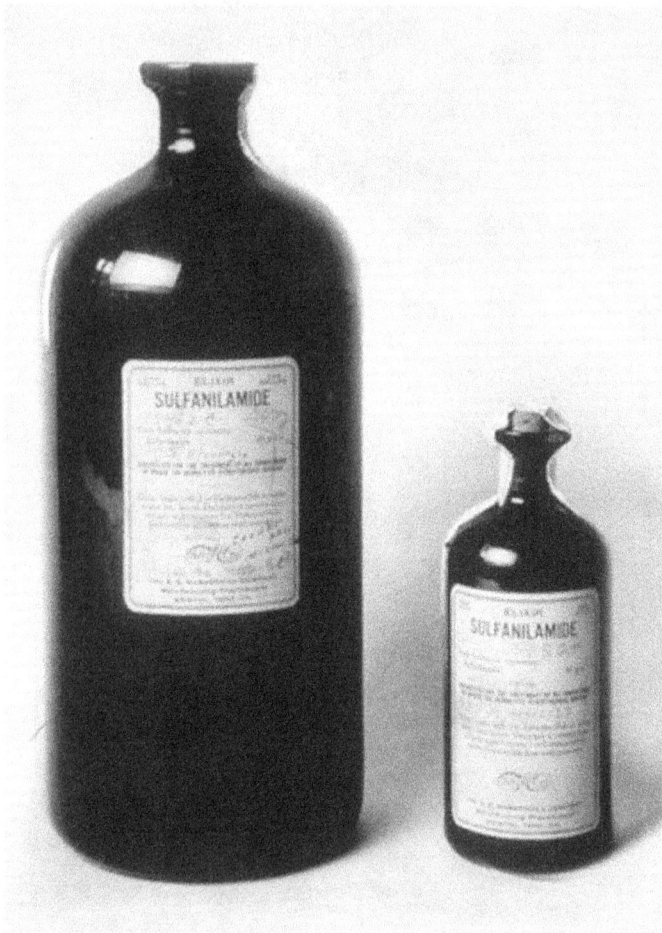

Figure 8.2. Elixir sulfanilamide bottles recovered by FDA in 1937. (Source: Wikimedia commons/FDA)

Elixir sulfanilimide deaths

Reports of the first six suspicious deaths arrived in the American Medical Association's (AMA) offices as early as 11 October from Tulsa, Oklahoma. (2) The Food and Drug Administration (FDA) was alerted and put in place the retrieval of all shipped bottles of the drug. Of the 240 gallons that had been shipped, 234 gallons and 1 pint were recovered. (5) However, the balance had been consumed and had caused the deaths of 107 people, mostly children. It is estimated that, had all the distributed 'elixir' been consumed, the death toll would have been around 4,500. (2) Those deaths had been slow and painful. The victims of elixir sulfanilimide poisoning would typically be ill for 7-21 days and would show features of renal failure including nausea, vomiting, convulsions and severe pain. (4)

One distraught and grieving mother, Maisie Nidiffer from Oklahoma, wrote to President Roosevelt himself to describe the death of her six-year old daughter, Joan.

> The first time I ever had occasion to call in a doctor for [Joan] and she was given Elixir of Sulfanilamide. All that is left to us is the caring for her little grave. Even the memory of her is mixed with sorrow for we can see her little body tossing to and fro and hear that little voice screaming with pain and it seems as though it drive me insane. ... It is my plea that you will take steps to prevent such sales of drugs that will take little lives and leave such suffering behind and such a bleak outlook on the future as I have tonight. (5)

With her letter, she enclosed a photograph of her now deceased child (fig. 8.3). Joan Nidiffer's smiling face made its way into numerous newspaper articles about the incident and even into the US Secretary of Agriculture's report. A face — that of a beautiful little girl — had been given to the tragedy.

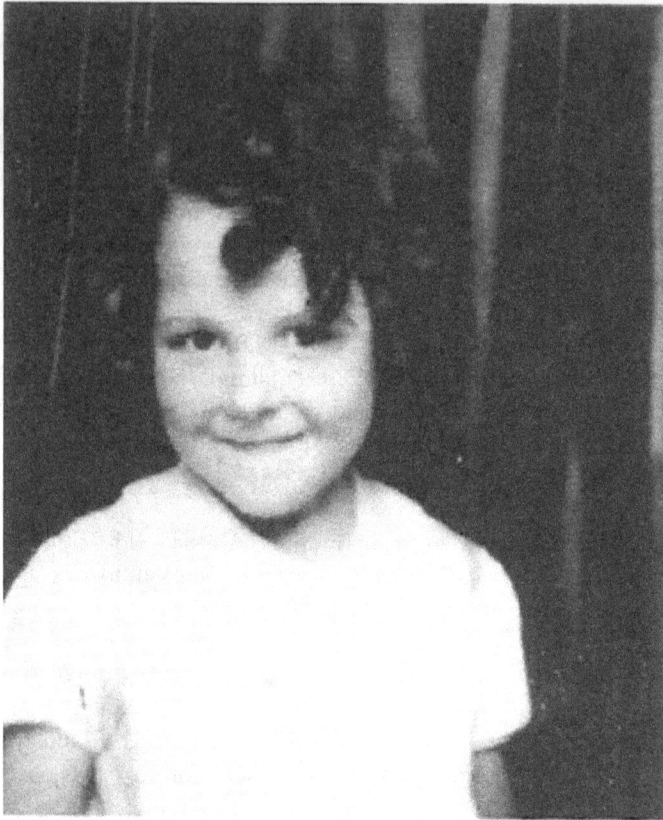

Figure 8.3. Joan Nidiffer. This photo was sent to President Roosevelt on 8 November 1937 by Maisie Nidiffer and is reproduced from the Report of the US Secretary of Agriculture, 1937.

Kelsey's supervisor, Eugene Geiling, was asked to be the principal academic pharmacologist consulting for the FDA and the AMA in the sulfanilimide affair. (2) As Geiling's graduate student, Kelsey helped conduct animal studies in rats, rabbits and dogs to find out which was the toxic element — the sulfanilamide itself or the solvent, diethylene glycol. (4) Kelsey later recalled, 'All graduate students were required to watch the progress of all these studies and to lend their assistance, wherever possible...' (6) Geiling later published these findings (7) showing conclusively that the solvent was the toxic agent, confirming a number of other earlier papers. Thus, the literature, even in 1937, could have been used to highlight the nephrotoxicity of diethylene glycol, but Massengill had been under no legal compulsion to investigate safety issues with their product.

Dr Samuel Evans Massengill, the company owner, said,

> My chemists and I deeply regret the fatal results, but there was no error in the manufacture of the product. We have been supplying a legitimate professional demand and not once could have foreseen the unlooked-for results. I do not feel that there was any responsibility on our part. (5)

While this may have been true from a strictly legal perspective, perhaps not all of Massengill's staff agreed with the abrogation of any moral responsibility. Indeed, the 108th death as a result of the sulphanilamide tragedy was the company pharmacist, Harold Watkins, who had proposed the use of diethylene glycol in the first place. He committed suicide in January 1939. (8)

New regulation — a focus on safety

Drugs at the beginning of the 20th century were almost completely unregulated. The US Pure Food and Drugs Act of

1906 had established penalties for the adulteration or misbranding of medicines, but by the 1920s this legislation was increasingly thought unfit for purpose. In the 1930s, the US Department of Agriculture (USDA) had joined forces with Senator Royal Copeland to sponsor new legislation to strengthen pharmaceutical regulation, but by 1937 this had failed to make it through Congress. Copeland's bill, although calling for reform, did not include any provisions for pre-marketing checks or for any form of federal licensing. (2)

The only charge that could be brought against Massengill, under the law at the time, was one of misbranding. They had labelled their product an 'elixir', when in fact it contained no alcohol. For this they were fined a total of US$26,100. (3,4) If they had called their product a 'preparation' or a 'solution' they would have committed no crime at all, despite the death toll. The powerlessness of the Federal Government to act, other than on the basis of such a trivial matter, was used in the argument to force through tougher legislation to control the future manufacture and sales of drugs.

When Copeland was asked if his proposed bill would have prevented the sulfanilimide tragedy, he said no, and that,

> ...the bill...should be amended to require a licence from the Government preliminary to the distribution of all drugs containing any potent ingredient or combination of ingredients, the use of which has not become well established in medical practice.

> In the interests of safety, society has required that physicians be licensed to practice the healing art. Pharmacists are licensed to compound drugs. Even steam-fitters, electricians and plumbers are required to have licenses. Certainly a requirement that potent proprietary medicines be manufactured under license can be justified on the ground of public safety. (9)

The US Secretary of Agriculture Henry A. Wallace produced a report on the tragedy. (10) This report included the Niddifer letter and the photo of Joan Niddifer and made four recommendations that form the basis of modern pharmaceutical regulation throughout the world:

> License control of new drugs to insure that they will not be generally distributed until experimental and clinical tests have shown them to be safe for use...
>
> Prohibition of drugs, which are dangerous to health when administered in accordance with the manufacturer's directions for use...
>
> Requirement that drug labels bear appropriate directions for use and warnings against probable misuse....
>
> Prohibition of secret remedies by requiring that labels fully disclose the composition of the drugs...(10)

Wallace's report very much framed the sulfanilimide affair as an avoidable tragedy, and one that needed a change in the law to ensure it could not recur. (2) Based on the report, Senator Copeland, redrafted his bill with the pre-marketing provisions, and after some political horse trading, the bill passed through Congress and President Roosevelt signed it into law on 25 June 1938, eight months after the first 'elixir' deaths. (11)

The US Federal Food, Drug, and Cosmetics Act of 1938 has been described as 'one of the most important regulatory statutes in American and perhaps global history.' (2) It created a new legal category — the 'new drug' — and authorised the FDA to serve as gatekeepers for such compounds entering the market place.

Thus, the FDA, which had emerged from the USDA's Bureau of Chemistry, first as a separate agency called the Food, Drug, and Insecticide Administration, and later shortened to the FDA in 1930 (12), had now acquired greater status and considerably sharper teeth, with pharmaceutical companies compelled to work in a new landscape of greater scrutiny and transparency. The new legislation had installed '...a regulatory sentry at the border between drug development and market...' and that sentry was the FDA. (2)

Kelsey's involvement in the 1938 legislative reform was obviously peripheral, but she was at the centre of the laboratory work that confirmed the toxicity of the 'elixir'. Twenty-five years later, when addressing the Medical Alumni Association of the University of Chicago, Kelsey said,

> The urgency of the situation, the intensive round-the-clock toxicologic studies and the subsequent changes in the law relative to the control of drugs could not and did not fail to make a deep impression on a graduate student such as myself in the University's Department of Pharmacology. (13)

It would be good to say that the elixir sulfanilimide tragedy, as well as ensuring the passage of new, tougher legislation, also ensured that we would avoid future cases of diethylene glycol poisoning. However, that would not be so, and, as the philosopher Hegel once remarked, 'the only thing we learn from history is that we learn nothing from history.' Many times over the last 50 years diethylene glycol has hit the headlines in association with drug related deaths. Unlike the pharmacist from Massengill, these modern drug manufacturers know exactly just how toxic diethylene glycol is, but because it is cheaper than glycerine it is being used as an alternative additive to turn a profit at the expense of lives.

Children die slowly from renal failure in exactly the same way as Joan Nidiffer did in Tulsa, Oklahoma in 1937. Occasional lives can now be saved through modern medical intervention, but in most of the communities where these adulterated drugs have been peddled no such care has been available, such as Bangladesh (14) and Haiti (15). Most recently, in 2013, two Nigerians were sentenced to seven years in prison over the deaths of at least 80 children who took an adulterated teething medicine containing diethylene glycol. (16)

That criminal charges can be brought at all is a consequence of the legislative journey that began in the US, largely as a result of the passing of the new Food, Drug, and Cosmetic Act. However, it would not end there and throughout the 20th and into the 21st centuries this legislation, which strives to create an environment that puts patient and public safety at the forefront, would be amended many times after its enactment.

One of the most important legislative changes would come in 1962, and this time Frances Kelsey would play the starring role. This is where the second act of her story begins.

Effectiveness, not just safety

In the late 1950s and early 60s, a Democratic Senator from Tennessee, Estes Kefauver, was acquiring quite a name for himself (fig. 8.4). He was the Chair of a Sub-Committee investigating Anti-Trust and Monopolies, and he was seen as a champion of the people, tackling organised crime and big business. Inevitably his attention turned to some of the biggest businesses of all — the pharmaceutical industry. Why were drugs so expensive? And, how could companies justify profits of 1000% or more? His Sub-Committee heard about these alleged price hikes, but they also heard evidence of mis-advertising, unsubstantiated claims and serious questions over the effectiveness of some drugs. (17)

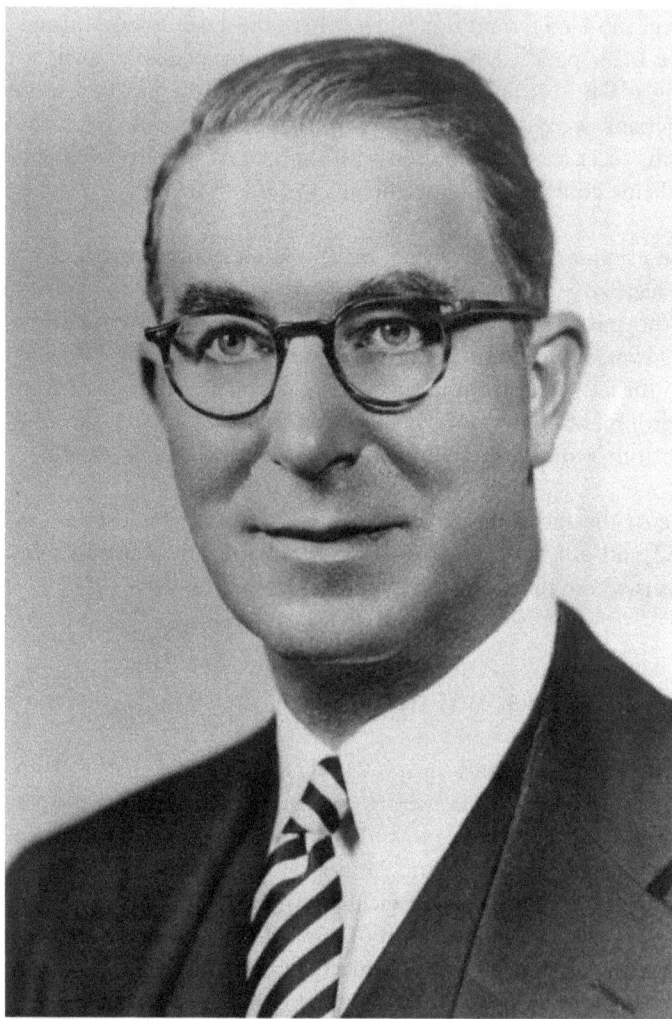

Figure 8.4. Senator Estes Kefauver, D-TN (1903-63) (Public Domain)

To rectify these, Kefauver proposed a range of new policies in the form of a bill in early 1961, which would amend the outdated 1938 Food, Drug, and Cosmetics Act. One of these reforms would require the US FDA to pass judgement on a drug's effectiveness, not just, as the 1938 Act required, its safety. However, Kefauver was viewed as a radical by many and received little support even from his own party, while his proposals irked both the medical profession in the form of the American Medical Association, and the pharmaceutical industry, in the form of the Pharmaceutical Manufacturers' Association. (2) Most importantly, perhaps, the public had little interest in drug regulatory reform, and without the necessary support Kefauver's bill languished in the committee rooms of Washington D.C.

Kelsey's journey to the FDA

In 1938, the same year that the new Federal Food, Drug, and Cosmetic Act was passed, Frances Kelsey obtained her PhD from the University of Chicago. She secured a job on the faculty and stayed in Chicago for the next twelve years. She also decided to study medicine and obtained her MD in 1950. (3,4)

For the next ten years she would work in a variety of jobs; as an editorial associate for the *Journal of the American Medical Association*, on the Pharmacology teaching staff at the University of South Dakota and as a general practitioner in the same state.

In 1960, the year that Senator Kefauver was assembling his doomed bill, Frances Kelsey's husband was offered a position at the National Institutes of Health in Washington D.C., and she began to look for job opportunities to enable her to join him. Geiling, Kelsey's former boss in Chicago, was now working at the FDA, and he proposed Kelsey for a job there. He described her as a 'brilliant' young student who could 'write so well'. (2) She was duly appointed as a medical officer and reviewer of new drug applications. (3,4,18)

In her first month on the job, Kelsey was assigned a new drug application to scrutinise. Kelsey later recalled, 'They gave it to me because they thought it would be an easy one to start on. As it turned out, it wasn't all that easy'. (4) The new drug application in question had been submitted to the FDA in September 1960 by the US pharmaceutical company Richardson-Merrell for their product, which was trade named *Kevadon*. The chemical name of their drug was thalidomide.

Thalidomide

Thalidomide had been developed in West Germany by the drug company Chemie Grünenthal GmbH, originally as an anticonvulsant, but its sedative properties were quickly identified. (19) The apparent safety of the drug was striking, for company scientists found that there was practically no dose that was lethal to rats. Given that other barbiturate based sedatives were lethal in overdose, the manufacturers and their licensees made much of their drug's safety. Indeed, in the UK one advertisement in the medical press showed a toddler with a bottle of the drug with the tagline, 'this child's life may depend on the safety of 'Distaval''. (fig. 8.5)

Thalidomide was launched in West Germany as *Contergan* in October 1957 and sold over-the-counter, without prescription. More than forty other countries followed including the UK, where the drug was launched in April 1958 as *Distaval*, by the British drug house Distillers, who had licensed the drug from the German manufacturers. As the drug also reduced nausea it became a popular sleeping tablet amongst pregnant women suffering from morning sickness.

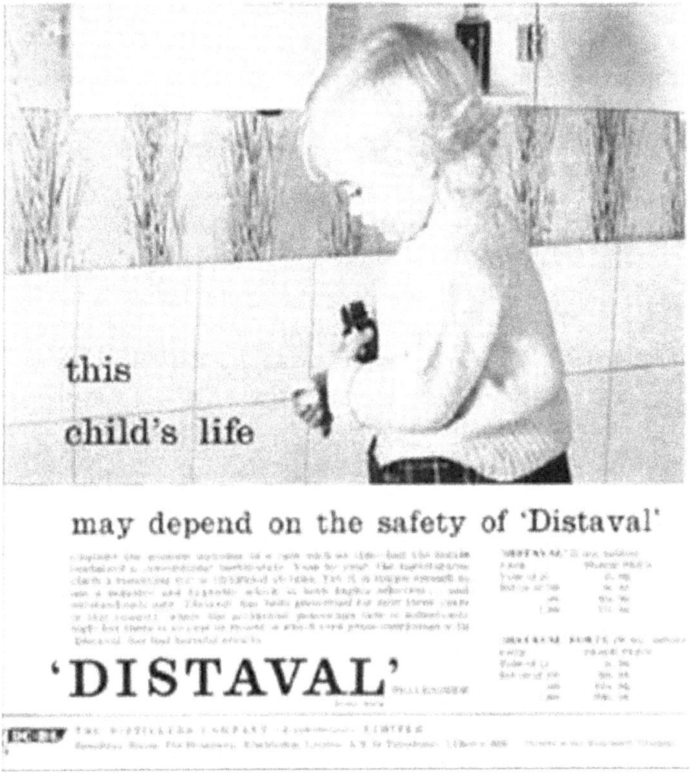

Figure 8.5. Distaval (thalidomide) advertisement, 1961. One of the main marketing strategies for thalidomide was to emphasise its safety in overdose. (Source: British Medical Journal, 24 June 1961)

The first thalidomide victim is thought to have been born in December 1956, before the drug was mass marketed. (20) The child's father was a Grünenthal employee in West Germany who had been given advanced samples of the sedative, which he had given to his pregnant wife. (21) However, it would be another five years before the link between the deformities and the drug would be made. (22, 23)

New Drug Application

When Kelsey studied the new drug application before her, she first looked at the quality of the supporting data. She immediately noted, 'the basic experimental work was inadequate. There were, for example, very little data regarding the absorption, distribution, metabolism, and excretion of the drug'. (24)

Kelsey responded to Merrell for the first time on 10 November 1960 stating that their application was incomplete. (25) At the time, the FDA had 60 days in order to deal with a new drug application, and a pharmaceutical company could go ahead with marketing their product if they heard nothing by this deadline. However, the deadline did not apply if the application was deemed by the FDA to be incomplete. On day 58, Kelsey rejected the application as such, presenting Merrell with their first rejection in a battle that would go on between them for 18 months. In her letter to the company, she noted that their application failed to report animal and clinical studies adequately and that many of the clinical cases presented were in summary form without the necessary detail she required. Overall, she felt there were inadequate numbers of cases and noted that many of those submitted were in foreign (non-US) literature. She added that some of the submission had been poorly translated from the original German and concluded, somewhat presciently, 'We feel that the side effects are passed over too lightly in the brochure'. (25)

In addition to her close reading of the application, Kelsey undertook a detailed literature review and took special note of any papers cited by Merrell. She also found a letter published in December 1960 by a Scottish General Practitioner in the BMJ, describing peripheral neuropathy in four of his patients taking thalidomide, with the title, 'Is thalidomide to blame?' (26)

She consulted others at the FDA, her former colleagues and other experts, including her husband. He responded in a formal memo and described one section of the Kevadon application as, 'an interesting collection of meaningless, pseudo-scientific jargon, apparently intended to impress chemically unsophisticated readers'. (27) Unfortunately for Merrell, Frances Kelsey with her 30 years of pharmacology experience was certainly not that.

Aside from her detailed and objective critique of the application, Kelsey also had two gut feelings to contend with. First, she felt the claims were too glowing — it was 'too good to be true' she remembered. Second, she was beginning to doubt the integrity of the company.

When the letter reporting the peripheral neuropathy had been published in the UK, it had prompted a response from Denis Burley, a Distillers official who noted that other such reports had been received in early 1960. (28) If this was indeed the case, why had Merrell neglected to include them in their application submitted several months later? Kelsey spoke with the recipient of her letter at Merrell, F. Joseph Murray, on 23 February 1961 and he failed to acknowledge the peripheral neuropathy reports until she confronted him with the BMJ letters. Later, investigative journalists at the *Sunday Times*, who spearheaded a campaign for thalidomide victims, pinpointed this as the likely moment when Merrell lost any chance of ever marketing their drug in the US. (2, 29)

In her notes of meetings at the FDA with officials from Merrell, Kelsey describes being pressurised and also tellingly on one occasion, 'I had the feeling throughout the day that they were at no time being wholly frank with me and that this attitude has obtained in all our conferences etc regarding this drug'. (30) Kelsey certainly had concerns based on the pharmacological deficiencies of the application, but almost from the start she also had doubts about the drug, because she had doubts about its sponsor. (2)

Merrell officials accused her of stubbornness, of simply avoiding making a decision and more. Of these company officials, Kelsey later told a *Life Magazine* reporter, 'Many of the things they called me you couldn't print'. (31)

These officials claimed that their application was experiencing, 'delay after delay after delay'. (2) She had requested further animal studies, including some looking at effects on the developing foetus, as well as longer term safety studies. Exasperated, senior staff at Merrell then went over her head and appealed to her bosses, including the FDA Medical Director. Her senior colleagues, however, gave Kelsey their full support.

Kelsey's main concern was that the peripheral neuropathy, that had first been reported in Scotland, might indicate a deeper level of toxicity. She was concerned that it may have foetal effects; the sedative had, after all, wide use amongst pregnant women suffering from morning sickness. This understanding of potentially adverse effects for the foetus had come from her work back in Geiling's laboratory in Chicago in the 1940s, where she had studied the effects of quinine on rabbits and their offspring. She was well aware that drugs could cross the placenta and of the markedly different pharmacological responses between adult and foetus that may ensue. These concerns of Kelsey predated any of the reports of teratogenicity from Europe, and she made them clear in her meetings with Merrell officials. (2)

Birth defects

Kelsey's concerns unfortunately proved to be justified as increased numbers of babies with a range of abnormalities were born in West Germany and in other countries where thalidomide had been sold. A striking feature of these abnormalities was phocomelia, which literally means seal extremities. These children had been born without the proper development of the long bones in their limbs, often giving their arms and/or legs a flipper like appearance. Sylvia Plath in her poem *Thalidomide* described this succinctly as 'knuckles at shoulder-blades'. (32)

Phocomelia was not unheard of before thalidomide, but it was very rare. One Danish study from 1949 estimated the frequency as approximately 1 in 800,000. (33) A much larger, more recent multinational study puts the estimate at 1 in 160,000. (34) By either reckoning, the condition would be so rare that most obstetricians would never encounter a single case in their professional lives. However, in West Germany alone, in the summer of 1960, there were 50-100 new cases a day. (2)

The mechanism of thalidomide's teratogenicity was unknown at the time, and was not revealed until 2010, when Japanese researchers found that the drug binds to the protein, cereblon. This protein when complexed with other regulators controls the expression of fibroblast growth factor 8, an essential regulator of limb development. (35)

In December 1961, two papers appeared from West Germany and Australia respectively linking the upsurge in these birth defects with thalidomide use in the first trimester of pregnancy. (22, 23) With this new intelligence, Chemie Grünenthal, the

German manufacturers, were forced to withdraw thalidomide from the European market on 27 November 1961. (36) In the US, however, Merrell continued to badger Kelsey with claims that there was no proof of a link. As the evidence grew and the full horror of the tragedy unfolded, Merrell 'quietly withdrew' the new drug application for Kevadon in March 1962. (2)

In April 1962, Helen B. Taussig, who had visited England and Germany to gather information about the epidemic of phocomelia, presented her findings at the Annual Meeting of the American College of Physicians in Philadelphia and later published her findings in the medical press in June and the popular science press in August (37, 38), where she remarked, 'The one-third who are so deformed that they die may be the luckier ones'. However, all this failed to make much of a splash in the lay press. That would come the following month with an article above the fold on the front page of the *Washington Post*. (39)

Kelsey and the media

This article, carrying a prominent photo of Kelsey, declared her the 'Heroine of FDA' and this was when her life changed irrevocably and the American public woke up to what had been happening. The article, which elevated Kelsey to virtual civic sainthood, was engineered by Kefauver — an astute political move that served to raise the temperature of the debate and to create a public appetite for change. (2) Now events shifted gear.

Three days later Kefauver introduced Kelsey and some of her FDA colleagues on the floor of Congress. Two weeks later, on 29 July 1962, the FDA announced that thalidomide had been available to American patients 'on an experimental basis'. The FDA later found that more than 2.5 million thalidomide tablets had been distributed by Merrell to over 1,000 physicians, and that they had dispensed these to almost 20,000 patients including hundreds of pregnant women. (20, 31, 40) As a result of this and some importing of thalidomide from abroad, 17 children were born in the US with thalidomide associated deformities. (4, 17, 20)

President Kennedy himself stepped in at this point to take the press conference three days later, highlighting the dangers of thalidomide and the major role played by Kelsey. (41)

Momentum growing, two days later there was a call in Congress for Kelsey to be honoured for her work, and remarkably this was realised in less than a week, when Kennedy presented Kelsey with the Distinguished Federal Civilian Service Medal at a highly publicised ceremony in the White House on 7 August 1962.

At the ceremony, the President said, 'I know that we are all most indebted to Dr. Kelsey... I know you know how much the country appreciates what you have done'. (42)

The spotlight now turned on Kelsey as never before. She was lauded in print throughout the US in every conceivable publication from the *New York Times* to the *Reader's Digest* to *Good Housekeeping*. 'Every American family stands in debt to Frances Kelsey,' declared the *New York Herald Tribune* (43) and in December 1962 she was named one of the ten most admired women in the world in a Gallup Poll (44). And, finally, Kelsey became, quite literally, the poster girl of the US Civil Service.

Over this time there was a shift in the reporting of the thalidomide story from one of 'narrowly averted disaster' to one of 'bureaucratic triumph'. (2) However, the bureaucracy had a human face, that of Frances Kelsey, and it almost seemed for a while as if Kelsey was the FDA. She did not promote this notion. She was always anxious to reinforce the teamwork involved in anything she had achieved. Even when she was awarded her medal she took pains to remind reporters that, 'Many people must be nominated for this award'. (2)

Amendments

Meanwhile, the Kennedy administration was drafting a new bill that came to resemble Kefauver's original from 1961, but also had input from Oren Harris, a Democrat Congressman from Arkansas. On 4 October 1962, the bill passed through both the House and the Senate on the same day. This legislative speed was almost unheard of, and had last been seen when the US declared war on Japan in December 1941.

John F. Kennedy signed the so-called Kefauver-Harris Amendments into law on 10 October 1962, in the Oval Office, with Kelsey and Kefauver standing behind him (fig. 8.6). Afterwards, Kennedy symbolically handed the pen he had used to Kelsey.

The 1962 Kefauver-Harris Amendments contained three core provisions. They required,

> positive evidence of 'effectiveness' and 'safety' in the form of 'adequate and well-controlled investigations'

> the designation of a drug as an *Investigational New Drug* during its period of assessment, and authorised the FDA to nullify this status and therefore terminate further studies if they were concerned with patient safety or study quality

> the FDA to establish and enforce new procedures to protect the interests and rights of patients in clinical research.

Interestingly, although the 1962 Amendments required evidence of efficacy, there was not, and indeed never had been, any question over thalidomide's efficacy. It was an excellent sedative. Its safety, not to the user, but to the foetus, was what was in question.

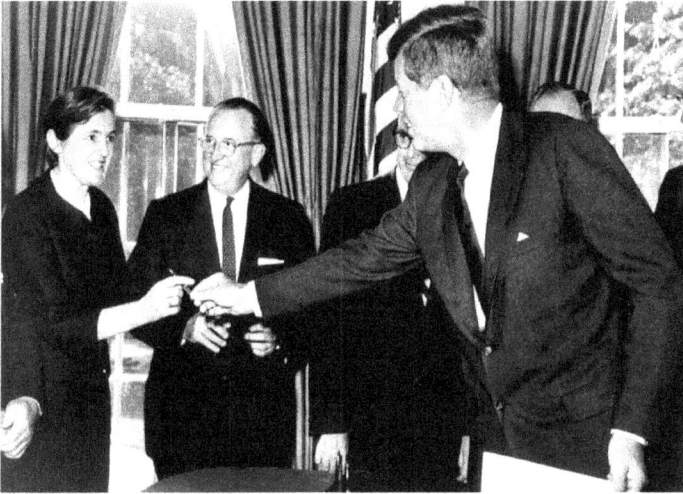

Figure 8.6. Frances Kelsey being offered the pen President John F. Kennedy had used to sign the Kefauver-Harris Amendments on 10 October 1963. (Source: FDA)

The proof of effectiveness requirement had been a central plank of Kefauver's original bill and had its origins in the lengthy hearings over which he presided. The thalidomide tragedy, although the result of a safety rather than an effectiveness issue, had put the regulation of drugs in general in play as it had not been since 1937. Circumstances had aligned to allow a major overhaul of the legislation.

The 1962 Amendments set the standard for evidentiary support for effectiveness relatively low in legal terms (40) by requiring *substantial evidence*, rather than *evidence beyond a reasonable doubt* or a *preponderance of evidence*. However, it went on to define this *substantial evidence* as,

Evidence consisting of adequate and well-controlled investigations, including clinical investigations, by experts qualified by scientific training and experience to evaluate the effectiveness of the drug involved, on the basis of which it could fairly and responsibly be concluded by such experts that the drug will have the effect it purports or is represented to have under the conditions of use prescribed, recommended, or suggested in the labeling or proposed labeling thereof. (45)

The use of the plural, 'investigations' is important and intentional, as is the emphasis placed on 'adequate and well-controlled' clinical trials, which would become the gold standard in all new drug evaluations.

Development of phased experimentation.

The 1962 Kefauver-Harris Amendments meant that the FDA had to issue regulations governing clinical experiments involving investigational drugs. This was especially important in that further clarification was needed on what constituted 'adequate and well-controlled' clinical trials. These rules, issued in 1963, included the need for informed consent, controlled experiments and for written study protocols. In addition, they also presented a new structure for drug research by defining a sequential, phased approach to clinical trials. (46)

From the 1950s there had been reference to Phase 1 and Phase 2 studies in the field of oncology and indeed the first published reference to a phased study was in 1960. (47) The phasing of clinical trials as we understand it today, however, was developed by the FDA. The notion of imposing three sequential phases of experiment to all investigational drugs was first discussed by the FDA in the Autumn of 1962. (48) Principal amongst the players in this discourse were Frances

Kelsey and her FDA colleague Julius Hauser. Each had different motives for pushing this agenda. Kelsey and the other Bureau of Medicine leaders wanted compulsory phased research in order to establish a prospective approach to trial design. Hauser and the other regulators wanted to curtail the increased use of experimentation as a means of marketing drugs before FDA approval. Both groups, however, wanted a 'rational', 'orderly' and 'comprehensive' approach to the testing of drugs. (48)

What started in 1963 as a controversial, bureaucratic and, to some, paternalistic approach to the conduct of clinical research had by the early 1970s become sufficiently mainstream to appear as the standard approach to drug testing in pharmacology textbooks. (48) And this approach, which started in Washington D.C., would soon spread to Europe, Japan and beyond, and persist largely unchanged in US legislation for over 50 years.

Originally, three phases were defined and these are laid out in the US Code of Federal Regulations (49),

> Phase 1 includes the initial introduction of an investigational new drug into humans. Phase 1 studies are typically closely monitored and may be conducted in patients or normal volunteer subjects. These studies are designed to determine the metabolism and pharmacologic actions of the drug in humans, the side effects associated with increasing doses, and, if possible, to gain early evidence on effectiveness.
>
> Phase 2 includes the controlled clinical studies conducted to evaluate the effectiveness of the drug for a particular indication or indications in patients with the disease or condition under study and to determine the common short-term side effects and risks associated with the drug. Phase 2 studies are typically well

controlled, closely monitored, and conducted in a relatively small number of patients, usually involving no more than several hundred subjects.

Phase 3 studies are expanded controlled and uncontrolled trials. They are performed after preliminary evidence suggesting effectiveness of the drug has been obtained, and are intended to gather the additional information about effectiveness and safety that is needed to evaluate the overall benefit-risk relationship of the drug and to provide an adequate basis for physician labeling. Phase 3 studies usually include from several hundred to several thousand subjects.

Since the original designation of Phase 1-3 trials, some groups have introduced a post-marketing Phase 4 and an early investigational or microdosing Phase 0. Although not universally recognised, these refinements have not changed the basic requirement in the FDA's original structure for a step-wise approach to drug testing and evaluation. This approach proceeds from safety to efficacy with progression to the next step contingent on the success of the last, and acts as a filter to remove unsafe or ineffective drugs from development and limit the exposure of human trial participants to undue risk.

While researchers also refer to studies involving non-pharmacological interventions, e.g. medical devices and psychological treatments, in terms of phases, this nomenclature was only ever intended to apply to drug studies.

In more recent years, the traditional phasing of studies has been criticised as a poor reflection of modern clinical research. (50) Many studies are now difficult to pigeon-hole as Phase 1, 2 or 3, and there is often blurring of the research goals between Phase 1/2 and 2/3. An alternative nomenclature of 'early phase' and 'late phase' is preferred by some and is gaining ground.

Conclusions

In 1937 and 1962, the emerging tragedies related to elixir sulfanilimide and thalidomide, respectively, opened the American public's eyes. Bills that had been stalled in Congress for years, were unexpectedly back on the table. Because of public outcry in both circumstances, suddenly the right thing to do coincided with the politically astute thing to do. This public outcry, however, is worthy of closer examination.

The public's perception of these tragedies had not been one of a complex bureaucracy wrangling with the intricacies of new legislation. Instead, these tragedies were personified and both were given a very visible face that helped crystallise the events in the minds of the public. In 1937, this had been the smiling face of six-year old Joan Niddifer, while in 1962 it was Frances Kelsey herself. Complex administrative debate had, in each case, been reduced to a single image. In 1937, the public wanted to avoid the loss of other 'little lives'. In 1962, they had been taught how the FDA in the form of a lone guardian had narrowly saved them from almost unimaginable tragedy.

The back room scenes of law making are rarely pretty and always byzantine. As Bismark is reputed to have said: there are two things you should never watch being made — laws and sausages. Kefauver, himself, on reviewing the passage of the Amendments said,

> ...those in the future who attempt to study the legislative history of this measure as it passed through its various stages may be forgiven if they become somewhat confused. (Quoted in ref 51)

The simple historical narratives of cause and effect that underpin Levine's phrase, 'born in scandal' (1) with which we began this chapter really do not do justice to the motives and machinations at work in Washington D.C. that midwifed the

1938 Food, Drug and Cosmetics Act and its 1962
Amendments. As well as suggesting that change can only be
enacted by the coercion of tragedy, the phrase also suggests
expediency and perhaps that of an inadequate and knee-jerk
response to circumstances. Kelsey, herself, was keen to point
out that this was not the case when she said,

> The thalidomide incident was a major factor leading to
> the enactment of the Kefauver-Harris Amendments of
> 1962. This has led to the conclusion by some that the
> law, and our investigational drug regulations, were
> hastily drawn and thus must have been poorly drawn.
> This is not correct. The Department's proposed
> legislation, which served as the basis for most of the
> provisions in the law as enacted which relate to drug
> testing, was very carefully drafted by experts and widely
> studied within the Executive Branch of the Government
> before it was sent to the Congress by our Secretary.
> Similarly the proposed investigational drug regulations
> were carefully prepared on the basis of many years of
> experience with the new drug law before the
> thalidomide situation came to public attention. (52)

Indeed, Kelsey had studied both recent UK and European
legislation and helped write FDA sponsored draft bills in 1960
and 1961 to reform drug regulation. (2) She was
corresponding with Geiling about the 1956 UK Therapeutic
Substances Act several months before thalidomide crossed her
desk. (53) Much thought over several years had indeed fed
into the drafting of the 1962 Amendments.

One 'thalidomider', as he prefers to be called, Randy Warren,
founder of the Thalidomide Victims Association of Canada
said, 'People pause today during pregnancy before they take a
tablet, before they smoke, before they take a drink, knowing
that it could possibly affect the fetus. Nobody knew that
before us.' (54) The reality is, however, that Kelsey did know

this and it was her concern, honed from years of research and study in pharmacology, that helped prevent a tragedy on an even greater scale.

Despite her experience, when Kelsey arrived in Washington D.C. in 1960, she was in a new job, at a new institution, in a new city and would undoubtedly have been anxious to get things right and make a good first impression. To take up a new post and be awarded the highest civilian honour by your President for your work before the end of your second year in the job is, by any standard, making an impression.

And what of the impact that Kelsey had on the reform of US drug regulation? Modern US legislation around drug development and testing, and by extension much of the derived legislation in other countries, owes a great debt to the work of Kelsey. Her role in the sulfanilimide tragedy was at the margins. Nevertheless, her meticulous approach to gathering and analysing the evidence was already being developed in the Chicago lab. And, she was able to see first hand the impact of pharmaceutical toxicity and the evidence needed to change the law to protect patients.

Sitting at her desk in the FDA almost 25 years later, she had learned enough and seen enough to have the courage of her convictions. She was up against powerful lobbying forces of the pharmaceutical industry, who were irritated by her delays, which they saw as nothing more than time wasting. Yet, she kept thalidomide out of the US and if that was all she had done in a long life of service, a generation of Americans would owe her a debt of gratitude. However, her resistance resulted in much more, for the thalidomide tragedy allowed the most radical overhaul of drug legislation the US had seen and, in turn, corresponding revisions of legislation around the world, including the UK.

After her initial work on thalidomide, Kelsey went on to be

appointed head of the new Investigational Drug Branch of the Bureau of Medicines and would work at the FDA for the next 42 years, retiring at the age of 90. (55) A decade before that retirement, Frances Kelsey would encounter thalidomide again because of renewed interest in its therapeutic potential in other diseases. She was invited to serve on the FDA's working Group to develop and implement uniform standards of safety for new clinical studies using thalidomide. Her experience with the drug was, of course, seen as a great advantage. (2) While she was acutely aware of the potential benefits that thalidomide may offer these patient groups, Kelsey was also understandably cautious. 'We need to take precautions,' she said, 'because people forget very soon'. (2)

—

That ability to neglect the lessons of the past, of which Kelsey was so well aware, is an appropriate point to conclude our journey through the history of drug research. This indeed is where we came in, with the hope that there might be some useful lessons to be learned by surveying the history of the subject. There have certainly been good stories of exceptional individuals and remarkable discoveries, but woven into those narratives there have also been themes and ideas that belong to no particular moment in history, but which resurface again and again across the centuries. There is the importance of observation, the relentless questioning and the meticulous attention to detail. Throughout our history, drugs have always been of high importance, and the quest for ever better treatments has in part driven the development of science. But, at the heart of it all there have always been patients, and the story of drug discovery is one of care as well as innovation; morality as well as entrepreneurial spirit. It has been a story of humanity, sometimes at its worst, but more often at its best.

References

1.   Carol Levine. Has AIDS changed the ethics of human subjects research? *Journal of Law, Medicine, and Ethics* 1988; 16: 3-4.

2.   Carpenter D. The ambiguous emergence of American pharmaceutical regulation, 1944-1961. Chap 3 in: *Reputation and Power Organizational Image and Pharmaceutical Regulation at the FDA*. Princeton University Press, Princeton, 2010.

3.   Biography, National Library of Medicine. https://www.nlm.nih.gov/changingthefaceofmedicine/physicians/biography_182.html (Accessed 10 January 2016).

4.   Bren L. Frances Oldham Kelsey: FDA Medical Reviewer Leaves Her Mark on History. *US Food and Drug Administration FDA Consumer Magazine*. March-April 2001.

5.   Ballentine C. Taste of raspberries, taste of death. The 1937 elixir sulfanilamide incident. *FDA Consumer Magazine* June 1981.

6.   Kelsey FO. From a speech 'Denial of Approval for Thalidomide in the United States', presented at the Medicine and Health Since World War II, National Library of Medicine, Bethesda, MD, 9 December 1993.

7.   Geiling EMK, Cannon PR. Pathologic effects of elixir of sufanilamide (diethylene glycol) poisoning. A clinical and experimental correlation: Final Report. *Journal of the American Medical Association* 1938; 111: 919-26.

8.   United Press. Chemist whose formula killed 67 kills himself. *Pittsburgh Press* 18 January 1939, Page 30.

9.	Letter, Campbell to Copeland, 29 October 1937; National Archives, Washington, D.C. and College Park, Maryland, RG 46, HR75A.

10.	U.S. Department of Agriculture, Report of the Secretary of Agriculture on Deaths Due to Elixir Sulfanilimide-Massengill, Submitted in Response to Senate Resolution 194 of November 16, 1937, Senate Document No. 124, 75th Congress, Second Session (Washington, D.C.: GPO).

11.	U.S. Food and Drug Administration FDA. http://www.fda.gov/RegulatoryInformation/Legislation/def ault.htm (Accessed 10 January 2016).

12.	U.S. Food and Drug Administration FDA. http://www.fda.gov/AboutFDA/WhatWeDo/History/Miles tones/ucm128305.htm (Accessed 10 January 2016).

13.	Kelsey FO. From a speech 'Chicago and New Drug Legislation' presented to the Medical Alumni Association, University of Chicago, 6 June 1963.

14.	Hanif M, Mobarak MR, Ronan A, Rahman D, Donovan JJ Jr, Bennish ML. Fatal renal failure caused by diethylene glycol in paracetamol elixir: the Bangladesh epidemic. *British Medical Journal* 1995; 311: 88-91.

15.	Bogdanich, W. FDA Tracked Poisoned Drugs, but Trail went cold in China. *New York Times*, 17 June 2007.

16.	BBC News Africa. My Pikin deaths: Nigerians jailed over poisoned baby drug. 17 May 2013. http://www.bbc.co.uk/news/world-africa-22574689#TWEET759279 (Accessed 10 January 2016).

17.	Goodrich WW. FDA Oral History Interview Transcript. 15-16 October 1986. http://www.fda.gov/downloads/AboutFDA/WhatWeDo/H

istory/OralHistories/SelectedOralHistoryTranscripts/UCM3 72999.pdf (Accessed 14 January 2016).

18. Hamburg MA. Commissioner of Food and Drugs — Remarks at the Award Ceremony for Dr. Frances Kelsey. http://www.fda.gov/NewsEvents/Speeches/ucm226349.htm (Accessed 10 January 2016).

19. Thalidomide. Exploring the history of medicine. Science Museum. London. www.sciencemuseum.org.uk/broughttolife/themes/controver sies/thalidomide.aspx (Accessed 10 January 2016).

20. Geraghty K. Profile of a role model. Protecting the public: Dr Frances Oldham Kelsey. *Virtual Mentor — American Medical Association Journal of Ethics.* November 2001. http://journalofethics.ama-assn.org/2001/11/toc-0111.html (Accessed 13 January 2016).

21. Rule A. The last German war secret, *Herald Sun* 27 June 2011. http://www.heraldsun.com.au/news/the-last-german-war-secret/story-e6frf7jo-1226082393923 (Accessed 10 January 2016).

22. McBride WG. Thalidomide and congenital abnormalities. *Lancet* 1961; 2: 1358.

23. Lenz W. Kindliche Missbildungen nach Mediakment wahrend der Graviditat. *Deutsche Medizinische Wochenschrift* 1961; 86: 2555-6.

24. Letter FOK to E. Iwarchiaha, Barcelona, Spain, 15 October 1962. (Quoted in Ref 2, Carpenter D. Reputation and Power, p217).

25. Letter: FOK to Wm S. Merrell Company ("Attention of Dr. Jos. Murray"), November 10, 1960. In Interagency Coordination in Drug Regulation and Research (ICDRR), 81.

26.   Florence AL. Is thalidomide to blame? [letter] *British Medical Journal* 1960; 2(5217): 1954.

27.   Memorandum: F.E. Kelsey to F.O. Kelsey, December 23, 1960. Subject: Comment on information concerning Kevadon submitted by Wm S. Merrell Co., December 9, 1960, in Interagency Coordination in Drug Regulation and Research (ICDRR), 85.

28.   Burley D. Is thalidomide to blame? [letter] *British Medical Journal* 1961; 1(5219): 130.

29.   Sunday Times Insight Team. *Suffer the Children: The Story of Thalidomide.* Viking Press, London, 1979.

30.   Kelsey F.O. Summary of Substance of Contact and Memo of Interview, March 30, 1961 Frances O. Kelsey Papers, Library of Congress, B1 (Quoted in Carpenter, *Reputation and Power* p221).

31.   Mulliken J. A woman doctor who would not be hurried. *Life* 1962; 53: L28-9.

32.   Plath S. Collected Poems. Faber & Faber, London, 2002.

33.   Birch-Jensen A. *Congenital deformities of the upper extremities.* Andelsbog trykkeriet, Odense, 1949.

34.   Bermejo-Sánchez E, Cuevas L, Amar E, Bianca S, Bianchi F, Botto LD, et al. Phocomelia: A worldwide descriptive epidemiologic study in a large series of cases from the International Clearinghouse for Birth Defects Surveillance and Research, and overview of the literature. *American Journal of Medical Genetics Part C (Seminars in Medical Genetics)* 2011; 157: 305-20.

35.   Ito T, Ando H, Suzuki T, Ogura T, Hotta K, Imamura Y, Yamaguchi Y, Handa H. Identification of a primary target of thalidomide teratogenicity. *Science* 2010; 327: 1345-50.

36.   Grünenthal Thalidomide Chronology. www.contergan.

grunenthal.info/grt-ctg/GRT-CTG/Die_Fakten/
Chronologie/152700079.jsp (Accessed 10 January 2016).

37.   Taussig HB. A study of the German outbreak of phocomelia. *JAMA* 1962; 180: 1106-24.

38.   Taussig HB. The thalidomide syndrome. *Scientific American* August, 1962.

39.   Mintz M. 'Heroine' of FDA Keeps Bad Drug Off of Market. *Washington Post* 15 July 1962.

40.   Temple R, Goldkind SF. The Food and Drug Administration and drug development. Historic, scientific , and ethical considertions. In: *The Oxford Textbook of Clinical Research Ethics.* Emanuel EJ, Lie RK, Grady C, Miller FG, Crouch RA, Wendler D (Eds). Oxford University Press, Oxford, 2008.

41.   The President's Press Conference of August 1, 1962 in Public Papers of the Presidents of the United States: John F. Kennedy, Containing the Public Messages, Speeches, and Statements of the President, 1961-1963 Washington D.C.: G.P.O., 1962-1964, Title 321.

42.   Kennedy JF. Remarks Upon Presenting the President's Awards for Distinguished Federal Civilian Service. August 7, 1962. www.presidency.ucsb.edu/ws/index.php?pid=8807 (Accessed 10 January 2016).

43.   Take warning from Thalidomide. *New York Herald Tribune*, 31 July 1962.

44.   Gallup G. Mrs Kennedy is most admired woman. *Washington Post*, 26 December 1962.

45.   U.S. Congress. Federal Food, Drug, and Cosmetic Act (codified in scattered sections of 21 U.S.C.; as amended through December 31, 2004. www.fda.gov/opacom/ laws/fdcact/fdctoc.htm (Accessed 10 January 2016).

46. FDA. Investigational New Drug Regulations under the Kefauver-Harris Amendments of 1963, reprint from CFR—Part 130, Section 130.3, August 1963.

47. Bethell FH, Louis J, Robbins A, Donnelly WJ, Dessel BH, Battle JD Jr, Pisciotta AV, Will J, Clifford GO. Phase II evaluation of cyclophosphamide. *Cancer Chemotherapy Reports* 1960; 8: 112-5.

48. Carpenter D. Reputation and power crystallized: Thalidomide, Frances Kelsey, and phased experimentation 1961-1966. Chap 4 in: *Reputation and Power Organizational Image and Pharmaceutical Regulation at the FDA.* Princeton University Press, Princeton, 2010.

49. CFR312.21. Code of Federal Regulations [Title 21, Volume 5] [Revised as of April 1, 2015].

50. Friedman LM, Furberg CD, DeMets DL. *Fundamentals of Clinical Trials.* 4th Edition. Springer, New York, 2010.

51. Brynner R, Stephens T. *Dark Remedy: The Impact of Thalidomide and its Revival as a Vital Medicine* Basic Books, Cambridge, MA, 2001.

52. Kelsey FO. Problems raised for the FDA by the occurrence of thalidomide embryopathy in Germany, 1960-61. Presented at the 91st Annual Meeting of the American Public Health Association, Kansas City, MO, November 14, 1963. In: Frances O Kelsey Papers, Library of Congress.

53. Letter: EMK Geiling to FO Kelsey, May 16, 1960. F Correspondence, K II. Eugene Maximilian Karl Geiling Papers, Johns Hopkins University, Baltimore.

54. Simpson JC. Pregnant pause. *Johns Hopkins Magazine* 53: 4 September 2001. www.jhu.edu/jhumag/0901web/pregnant.html (Accessed 10 January 2016).

55.   Sieff M. America's greatest living heroine Frances Oldham Kelsey – 98 and forgotten. *Baltimore Post Examiner*. 11 February 2013. http://baltimorepostexaminer.com/americas-greatest-living-heroine-frances-oldham-kelsey-98-and-forgotten/2013/02/11#sthash.N1tUfQZA.dpuf   (Accessed 10 January 2016).

—— ■ ——

Appendix

Nobel Prizes Awarded for Drug-related Research

Between 1901 and 2015, the Nobel Prize in Physiology or Medicine has been awarded to 210 laureates. It is a testament to the importance of drug related research that this prestigious prize has been awarded for major discoveries in pharmacology to no less than forty of these individuals. In addition, many others Nobel Prizes, especially in the fields of biochemistry, cell biology, immunology and molecular genetics, have been awarded for discoveries that have allowed modern drug research and new drug discovery to move forward.

A survey of those awards primarily for drug-related research provides an interesting timeline of discovery throughout the 20th and the early 21st centuries.

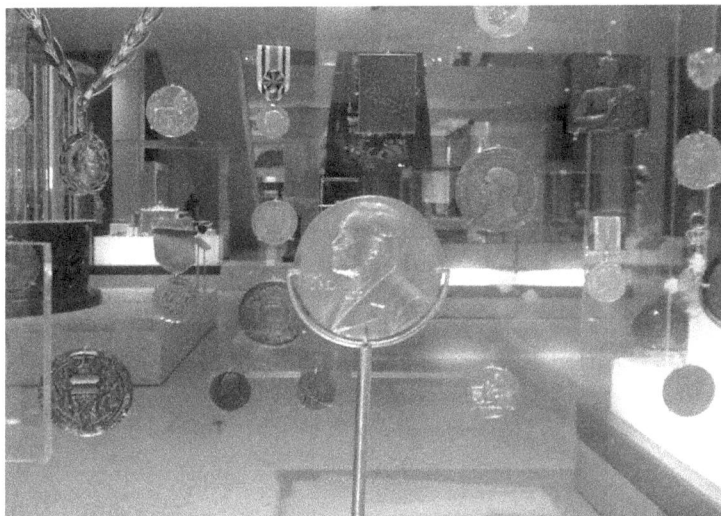

Sir Alexander Fleming's Nobel Prize medal along with his many other honours and awards on display in the National Museum of Scotland, Edinburgh. (Photo by the author)

2015
William C. Campbell and Satoshi Omura
'for their discoveries concerning a novel therapy against infections caused by roundworm parasites'

Youyou Tu
'for her discoveries concerning a novel therapy against Malaria'

2000
Arvid Carlsson, Paul Greengard and Eric R. Kandel
'for their discoveries concerning signal transduction in the nervous system'

1998
Robert F. Furchgott, Louis J. Ignarro and Ferid Murad
'for their discoveries concerning nitric oxide as a signalling molecule in the cardiovascular system'

1994
Alfred G. Gilman and Martin Rodbell
'for their discovery of G-proteins and the role of these proteins in signal transduction in cells'

1988
James W. Black, Gertrude B. Elion and George H. Hitchings
'for their discoveries of important principles for drug treatment'

1982
Sune K. Bergström, Bengt I. Samuelsson and John R. Vane
'for their discoveries concerning prostaglandins and related biologically active substances'

1971
Earl W. Sutherland, Jr.
'for his discoveries concerning the mechanisms of the action of hormones'

1970
Bernard Katz, Ulf von Euler and Julius Axelrod
'for their discoveries concerning the humoral transmittors in the nerve terminals and the mechanism for their storage, release and inactivation'

1966
Charles B Huggins
'for his discoveries concerning hormonal treatment of prostatic cancer'

1957
Daniel Bovet
'for his discoveries relating to synthetic compounds that inhibit the action of certain body substances, and especially their action on the vascular system and the skeletal muscles'

1952
Selman A Waksman
'for his discovery of streptomycin, the first antibiotic effective against tuberculosis'

1950
Edward C Kendall, Tadeus Reichstein and Philip S Hench
'for their discoveries relating to the hormones of the adrenal cortex, their structure and biological effects'

1948
Paul H Müller
'for his discovery of the high efficiency of DDT as a contact poison against several arthropods'

1945
Alexander Fleming, Ernst B Chain and Howard W Florey
'for the discovery of penicillin and its curative effect in various infectious diseases'

1943
Henrik CP Dam
'for his discovery of vitamin K'

Edward A Doisy
'for his discovery of the chemical nature of vitamin K'

1939
Gerhard Domagk
'for the discovery of the antibacterial effects of prontosil'

1936
Henry H Dale and Otto Loewi
'for their discoveries relating to chemical transmission of nerve impulses'

1923
Frederick G Banting and John JR Macleod
'for the discovery of insulin'

1908
Ilya I Mechnikov and Paul Ehrlich
'in recognition of their work on immunity'

—— ■ ——

INDEX

189

T

U

V

W

ABOUT THE AUTHOR

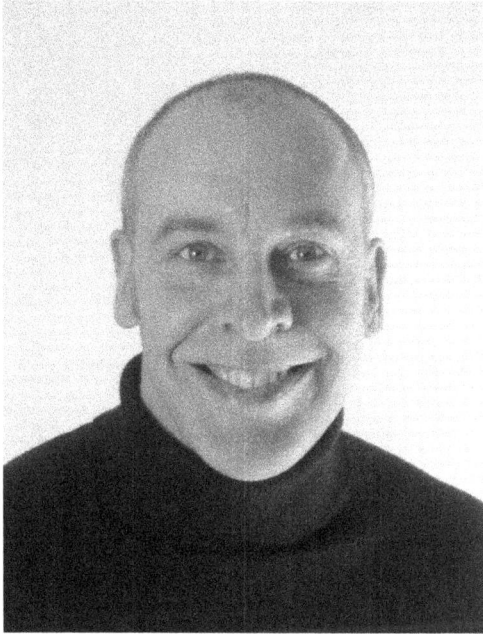

Allan Gaw, MD, PhD, FRCPath, FFPM, PGCert Med Ed is a Scottish writer and educator. He has been a clinical academic for over 25 years. Most recently he was Professor & Director of the Clinical Research Facility at Queen's University Belfast, and he previously worked at the University of Glasgow and UT Southwestern in Dallas, Texas.

In addition to over 25 books, he also writes and publishes articles on a range of subjects and a blog entitled *The Business of Discovery* (researchet.wordpress.com). This is his third book on the history of medical research.

If you would like to learn more about him and his work, visit his website www.allangaw.com or follow him on twitter @ResearchET.